Users' Guide to the Musculoskeletal Examination
Fundamentals for the Evidence-Based Clinician

Edited by
Timothy W. Flynn
Joshua A. Cleland
Julie M. Whitman

Cover art and illustrations by Mary E. McGivern

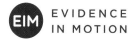

www.evidenceinmotion.com

Additional copies of this book may be ordered by calling 888 709-7096 or visiting the Web site at www.evidenceinmotion.com.

ISBN 978-0-9714792-3-4

To our professional colleagues who provided invaluable insight along the way, Dr. John Childs, Dr. Tony Delitto, Dr. Julie Fritz, Dr. Stephen Allison, Henry McCracking, and Dr. Rob Wainner.

TABLE OF CONTENTS

OVERVIEW

In This Chapter:

Introduction

The trend towards conscientious use of Evidence-Based Practice (EBP) continues to increase in the medical and healthcare professions. Sackett1 has defined EBP as an integration of the best available research evidence and clinical expertise with the patient's values. Experts in practice are often considered those clinicians who possess certain values, communication skills, decision-making processes, specialty certification, and years of practice.[2,3] A recent systematic review has shown that although it is expected that experienced physicians would have accumulated more knowledge and skills than their younger counterparts which should result in improved quality of care, this is not the case.[4] In fact Choudhry et al4 demonstrated that the amount of "experience" a physician possessed was inversely related to the quality care provided.[4] Although this systematic review leads one to question the association between experience and outcomes, researchers only included physicians in their studies and therefore the results cannot be directly extrapolated to other healthcare professionals.

The basic tenets of EBP are not intended to devalue "expertise". However, the point should be made that expertise alone is insufficient to assure optimal outcomes and hence the best available evidence should be incorporated into clinical decision-making.[4,5] It is essential to incorporate the best available evidence into each aspect of clinical decision-making from diagnosis, using tests and measures that posses the greatest degrees of reliability and validity possible, to prognosis of expected outcome based upon current literature and pattern recognition from clinical experience.[1]

One component of patient management that requires the incorporation of EBP is the diagnostic process. This entails gathering subjective information and objective data to develop an initial working hypothesis. Clinicians have a variety of specific tests and measures that can be used when determining the patient's initial diagnosis. The purpose of the tests and measures is to provide information to surpass the treatment threshold, the point in the examination process whereby the clinician feels confident that he/she can now begin treatment.[6] Traditionally, textbooks have disregarded information relative to the usefulness of a particular test or measure. This can cause clinicians to make incorrect treatment decisions.[7] Hence, the importance of understanding the diagnostic accuracy of a test or measure prior to incorporating it into clinical practice and using it to guide decision-making should not be underestimated.[8] Although the volume and quality of emerging evidence in the area of diagnostic utility of the clinical examination is emerging, there are still many areas where evidence is sparse. However, rather than waiting for the "perfect evidence", clinicians follow the approach advocated by Reinertsen[9] who suggests that clinicians should act on the research evidence that is available, and that they use patient-centered outcome tools to guide clinical decision-making.

This text will guide clinicians through the musculoskeletal examination while incorporating the evidence. This chapter will discuss the properties of reliability, sensitivity, specificity and likelihood ratios and the remainder of the text will guide the clinician through the musculoskeletal examination from ruling out red flags, through patient observation, palpation, range of motion assessment, joint assessment and special tests.

Reliability

Reliability is consistency of a measurement.[10] Intra-examiner reliability is the consistency of measurements between one person. Inter-examiner reliability is the consistency of measurements between two or more people.[10] The following scale is often used to determine the strength of the coefficients when calculating reliability: 0.50 represents poor reliability, 0.50-0.75 represents moderate reliability, and greater than 0.75 represents good reliability.[10]

Diagnostic Accuracy

Diagnosis:

Obtaining an accurate diagnosis for patients with musculoskeletal disorders relies on astute clinical reasoning skills of the clinician and careful analysis of data collected during the patient history and physical examination. Prior to beginning the examination the therapist determines the likelihood (pretest probability) that the patient presents with a specific disorder (e.g., adhesive capsulitis, shoulder impingement, etc). Pretest probability is based on the patient's past medical history and clinician experience.[11] The clinician then obtains a history from the patient to further ascertain the presence of a clinical condition. The therapist must subsequently identify tests and measures with adequate diagnostic accuracy that can provide information that assists with identifying the likelihood that a patient presents with a specific shoulder disorder following the examination (posttest probability).

Prior to identifying the tests and measures that posses the best diagnostic utility, the clinician must understand the properties of diagnostic accuracy which is often expressed in terms of sensitivity and specificity, and likelihood ratios (LRs).[1,12]

Sensitivity

Sensitivity is defined as the ability of a test to identify patients that have a particular disorder.[1] Highly sensitive tests are good for ruling **out** a specific diagnosis. The acronym "**SnNout**" can be used to remember that a test with high **S**ensitivity and a **N**egative result is good for ruling out the disorder.[1] An example comes from Walton and colleagues[13] who identified that palpation of the acromioclavicular (AC) joint exhibited a sensitivity of 0.96 for identifying the presence of AC joint lesions. Since the test has high sensitivity it is very likely to capture the majority of patients with AC joint involvement. However, it is also likely to capture a multitude of patients who do not have the disorder. Yet, if the test is **negative** we can be fairly confident that the patient does **NOT** have AC joint involvement.

Specificity

Specificity is defined as the ability of a test to identify patients that do not have a particular disorder.[1] Highly specific tests are good for ruling **in** a disorder. The acronym "**SpPin**" can be used to remember that a test with high **S**pecificity and a **P**ositive result is good for ruling in the disorder.[1] The crank test, as investigated by Liu et al,[14] provides an example of this. The authors identified the test as being highly specific (0.93). Since the test has high specificity a negative test finding would likely capture the majority of those without a labral tear. So in this case a **positive** test would be good for identifying all those **WITH** a labral tear

Likelihood Ratios

Although sensitivity and specificity are helpful there are a few limitations to these statistics.[11,15,16] Hence, likelihood ratios (LRs) are often the most clinically useful tool for determining shifts in probability if a patient presents with a specific disorder. Likelihood ratios are calculated by incorporating both the sensitivity and specificity and can directly alter the likelihood that the disorder is present.[17] Likelihood ratios are either positive (+LR) or negative (-LR). If a test is positive, then the +LR is used to determine the increased likelihood that a patient presents with the disorder of interest. Conversely, if a test is found to be negative, then the –LR is used to indicate a shift in the probability that the patient does not have the disorder. Table 1 provides a guide to interpreting LRs.[18]

Positive Likelihood Ratio	Negative Likelihood Ratio	Interpretation
Greater than 10	Less than 0.1	Generate large and often conclusive shifts in probability
5-10	0.1-0.2	Generate moderate shifts in probability
2-5	0.2-0.5	Generate small but sometimes important shifts in probability
1-2	0.5-1	Alter probability to a small and rarely important degree

Table 1. Interpretation of likelihood ratios. [18]

SUMMARY

Clinicians should be aware of the reliability, sensitivity, specificity and likelihood ratios of a particular test prior to incorporating it into clinical practice. Recently there has been a significant increase in the number of studies investigating the diagnostic utility of tests and measures used in the clinical setting. Each of the respective chapters in this User's Guide will list special tests and their diagnostic values where appropriate.

Reference List

(1) Sackett DL, Straws SE, Richardson WS et al. Evidence-Based Medicine; *How to Practice and Teach EBM*. 2nd ed. London: Harcourt Publishers Limited, 2000.

(2) Jensen GM, Gwyer J, Shepard KF. Expert practice in physical therapy. *Phys Ther* 2000;80:28-43.

(3) Shepard KF, Hack LM, Gwyer J et al. Describing expert practice in physical therapy. *Qual Health Res* 1999;9:746-58.

(4) Choudhry NK, Fletcher RH, Soumerai SB. Systematic review: the relationship between clinical experience and quality of health care. *Ann Intern Med* 2005;142:260-73.

(5) Whitman JM, Fritz JM, Childs JD. The influence of experience and specialty certifications on clinical outcomes for patients with low back pain. *J Orthop Sports Phys Ther* 2004;11-662.

(6) Kassirer JP. Our stubborn quest for diagnostic certainty a cause of excessive testing. *NEJM* 1989;320:1489-91.

(7) Bossuyt PMM. The quality of reporting in diagnostic test research: Getting better, still not optimal. *Clin Chem* 2004;50:465-7.

(8) Lijmer JG, Mol BW, Heisterkamp S et al. Empirical evidence of design-related bias in studies of diagnostic tests. *AMA* 1999;282:1061-963.

(9) Reinertsen JL. Zen and Art of Physican Autonomy Maintenance. *Ann Intern Med* 2003;138:992-5.

(10) Portney LG, Watkins MP. Foundations of Clinical Research: Applications to Practice. 2nd ed. Upper Saddle River: *Prentice Hall Health*, 2000.

(11) Bernstein J. Decision analysis (Current concepts review). *J Bone Joint Surg Am* 1997;79:1404-14.

(12) McGinn T, Guyatt G, Wyer P et al. Users' guides to the medical literature XXII: How to use articles about clinical decision rules. *JAMA* 2000;284:79-84.

(13) Walton J, Mahajan S, Paxinos A et al. Diagnostic values of tests for acromioclavicular joint pain. *J Bone Joint Surg Am* 2004;86-A:807-12.

(14) Liu SH, Henry MH, Nuccion SL. A prospective evaluation of a new physical examination in predicting glenoid labral tears. *Am J Sports Med*. 1996;24:721-5.

(15) Boyko EJ. Ruling out or ruling in disease with the most sensitive or specific diagnostic test: Short cut or wrong turn? *Med Decis Making* 1994;14:175-80.

(16) Riddle DL, Stratford PW. Interpreting validity indexes for diagnostic tests: An illustration using the berg balance test. *Phys Ther* 1999;79:939-48.

(17) Hayden SR, Brown MD. Liklihood ratio: A powerful tool for incorporating the results of a diagnostic test into clinical decision making. *Ann Emerg Med* 1999;33:575-80.

(18) Jaeschke R, Guyatt GH, Sackett DL. Users' guides to the medical literature. III. How to use an article about a diagnostic test. B. What are the results and will they help me in caring for my patients? The Evidence-Based Medicine Working Group. *JAMA* 1994;271:703-7.

SELF-REPORT INSTRUMENTS

The following self-report measures can be found on the CD accompanying this User's Guide.

> Medical Screening Form
> Patient Specific Functional Scale
> Numeric Pain Rating Scale
> Neck Disability Index (NDI)
> Quick Disability of the Shoulder Arm and Hand (DASH)
> Oswestry Disability Index (ODI)
> Lower Extremity Functional Scale (LEFS)
> Global Rating of Change
> Fear-Avoidance Beliefs Questionnaire

Psychometric Properties of Self-Report Measures

There has been an increasing trend in the use of outcome measures that capture a patient's current level of function, activities and participation, and disability. This is often accomplished through the use of self-report measures to capture data regarding a patient's perceived level of disability and the impact of a disease on a patient's daily activities.[1] It is essential for clinicians to use self-report measures that possess the characteristics of reliability and validity, and are responsive enough to identify changes in function when a true change has occurred.[1]

Reliability is the degree of consistency to which an instrument or rater measures a particular attribute.[2] When the reliability of a measurement is investigated, an attempt is made to determine the proportion of the measurement that is a true representation of the measure and the proportion that is the result of measurement error.[3] Measurements can be effected by error, which is a deviation from the true measurement as a result of chance.[3] It has been reported that reliability values closer to 1 exhibit higher levels of reliability.[6] "Acceptable reliability" has been reported to be values over .70, however, the individual clinician must determine the extent of reliability necessary to use the instrument in clinical practice.[4]

Test-retest reliability is the ability of a questionnaire to repeatedly capture similar scores on two separate occasions of test administration, over which time the patient has not exhibited a change in their condition.[3] When using self-report outcome measures it is important to know the minimal detectable change (MDC), the amount of change that must be observed before the change can be considered to exceed the measurement error.[5] For example if the measurement error for a particular outcome tool is 4 points, any changes in scores lower than 4 can only be attributed to error and not a true change in patient status.

Validity is the extent to which an instrument measures exactly what it is intended to measure.[3] In addition, functional and disability level measures must be able to detect a change when a true change has occurred and must remain stable when one has not.[5] Responsiveness, the ability of a test or measure to recognize change[3], is essential in detecting a clinically meaningful level of change.[6] This clinically meaningful level of change is often referred to as the minimal clinically important difference (MCID), the smallest difference which indicates a true change in the patients functional abilities, activities and participation, or level of disability has occurred.[7] Specific values for the reliability, MDC and MCID for specific outcome measures presented on this text can be found in the Table.

Outcome Tool	Reliability	Minimal Clinically Important Difference
Neck Disability Index	50 - .68[8,9]	7% - 19%[8,9]
Quick Dash	.90[10]	Not reported
Oswestry Disability Index	.90[11]	6%[11]
Lower Extremity Functional Scale	.98[12]	8-9 points[6,12]
Global Rating of Change	Not reported	• Scores on the GRC between ±3 and ±1 represent small changes[7] • Scores between ±4 and ±5 represent moderate changes[7] • Scores of ±6 or ±7 large changes[7]
Numeric Pain Rating Scale	.76[8]	2 points[8,9,13]
Patient Specific Functional Scale	.82- .92[8,14]	2.0[8]
Fear-Avoidance Beliefs Questionnaire: Physical Activity Subscale	Back pain : .77[15] Neck pain : .85[16]	Not reported
Fear-Avoidance Beliefs Questionnaire: Work Subscale	Back pain: .90[15] Neck pain: .93[16]	Not reported

Reference List

(1) Pietrobon R, Coeytaux R, Carey T et al. Standard scales for measurement of functional outcome for cervical pain or dysfunction. *Spine* 2002;27:515-22.

(2) Rothstein JM, Echternach JL. Primer on Measurement: An Introductory Guide to Measurement Issues. Alexandria, VA: *American Physical Therapy Association*, 1999.

(3) Portney LG, Watkins MP. Foundations of Clinical Research: Applications to Practice. 2nd ed. Upper Saddle River: *Prentice Hall Health*, 2000.

(4) Wainner RS. Reliability of the clinical examination: how close is "close enough"? *J Orthop Sports Phys Ther* 2003;33:488-91.

(5) Resnik L, Dobrzykowski E. Guide to outcomes measurement for patients with low back pain syndromes. *J Orthop Sports Phys Ther* 2003;33:307-16.

(6) Binkley JM, Stratford PW, Lott SA et al. The Lower Extremity Functional Scale (LEFS): scale development, measurement properties, and clinical application. North American Orthopaedic Rehabilitation Research Network. *Phys. Ther.* 1999;79:371-83.

(7) Jaeschke R, Singer J, Guyatt GH. Measurment of health status: Ascertaining the minimal clinically important difference. *Controlled Clinical Trials* 1989;10:407-15.

(8) Cleland JA, Fritz JM, Whitman JM et al. The reliability and construct validity of the Neck Disability Index and Patient Specific Functional Scale in patients with cervical radiculopathy. *Spine* 2006;31:598-602.

(9) Cleland JA, Childs JD, Whitman JM. Psychometric properties of the neck disability index and numeric pain rating scale in patients with mechanical neck pain. *Arch Phys Med Rehab.* 2008; In Press.

(10) Gummesson C, Ward MM, Atroshi I. The shortened disabilities of the arm, shoulder and hand questionnaire (QuickDASH): validity and reliability based on responses within the full-length DASH. *BMC Musculoskeletal Disorders* 2006;7:44.

(11) Fritz JM, Irrang JJ. A comparison of a modified Oswestry Low Back Disability Questionnaire and the Quebec Back Pain Disability Scale. *Phys Ther* 2001;81:776-88.

(12) Watson CJ, Propps M, Ratner J et al. Reliability and responsiveness of the lower extremity functional scale and the anterior knee pain scale in patients with anterior knee pain. *J Orthop Sports Phys Ther* 2005;35:136-46.

(13) Childs JD, Piva SR, Fritz JM. Responsiveness of the numeric pain rating scale in patients with low back pain. *Spine* 2005;30:1331-4.

(14) Westaway M, Stratford P, Binkley J. The Patient-Specific Functional Scale: validation of its use in persons with neck dysfunction. *J Orthop Sports Phys Ther* 1998;27:331-8.

(15) Jacob T, Baras M, Zeev A et al. Low back pain: reliability of a set of pain measurement tools. *Arch Phys Med Rehabil* 2001;82:735-42.

(16) Cleland JA, Childs JD, Fritz JM. The Psychometric Properties of the Fear-Avoidance Beliefs Questionnaire and the Tampa Scale of Kinesiophobia in Patients with Neck Pain. *Am J Phys Med Rehab* 2007; In Press.

Self-Report

Medical Screening Examination

In This Chapter:

Medical Screening Examination

Clinical decision-making requires a detailed history and physical examination to determine if the patient's symptoms are systemic or musculoskeletal in origin. During the time of the examination the clinician should take a thorough history and perform a systems review. Once the examination is complete the clinician then must determine if the patient presents with musculoskeletal impairments and treatment can begin, or if the patient exhibits other findings and requires a consultation with or referral to another healthcare professional. In this chapter we discuss common red flags and signs or symptoms that suggest a more serious underlying pathology that may necessitate a referral for medical interventions. We will outline the medical screening process including the historical examination, and identification of referral patterns and signs and symptoms of systemic disease.

Prior to initiating the examination the clinician should carefully review the medical intake questionnaire to determine if the patient has previously been diagnosed with any systemic disease that may be contributing to current symptoms. Following a review of the intake questionnaire the clinician should begin the historical examination by asking the patient to further elaborate on any disease experienced in the past and to clarify items on the intake questionnaire.

Questions might include:

1. *When were you diagnosed with the particular disease?*
2. *How was it treated?*
3. *Is it currently being treated?*
4. *Are the symptoms you are experiencing today different than when you were first diagnosed with the disorder?*
5. *Are you taking any medications for this current condition or any other diagnoses?*

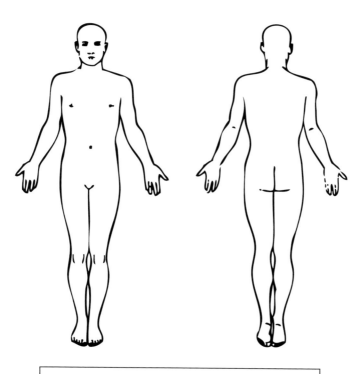

///	Stabbing	XXX	Burning
000	Pins & Needles	===	Numbness

Pain Diagram

Once data related to the past medical history have been obtained the clinician should begin questioning the behavior of the current symptoms to investigate if they are related to the musculoskeletal system or are presenting as non-musculoskeletal in nature. The following general questions should be asked to initially identify the possibility of symptoms that are constitutional and require referral to another medical professional:[1]

1. *Have you experienced any unexplained weight loss or gain greater than 10 pounds?*
2. *Have you experienced a fever, sweating at night, or chills?*
3. *Have you experienced a loss of appetite or nausea and/or vomiting?*
4. *Have you experienced any dizziness or diarrhea?*
5. *Are you awakened with pain at night? If so, does it resolve quickly with changes in position or does it keep you awake?*

The clinician should also question the patient regarding current medication usage. A number of side effects can occur with the use of individual medications or combinations of medications. A detailed description of the side effects associated with various medications is beyond the scope of this User's Guide.

Additionally there are a number of questions that indicate pathology of a specific system. Specific questions relative to each system and referral patterns of each system will be described in detail in the following pages.

Cardiovascular System

There are a number of risk factors associated with disease of the cardiovascular system. When questioning the patient the clinician should be sure to ask specific questions related to risk factors including:[2]

1. *Do you have a family history of cardiovascular disease?*
2. *What is your diet?*
3. *Do you have a history of smoking?*
4. *What are your current and recent levels of stress?*
5. *Do you have a history of diabetes?*

Follow-up questions to ascertain the possibility that the patient may be presenting with symptoms associated with cardiovascular disease include the following:[1,3]

1. *Do you experience any difficulty breathing?*
2. *Do you experience an increase in chest pain with increased exertion?*
3. *Have you been experiencing any heart palpitations, tachycardia, bradycardia, nausea, diaphoresis, or chest pressure?*
4. *Have you experienced episodes of syncope?*
5. *Do you ever experience excessive fatigue?*

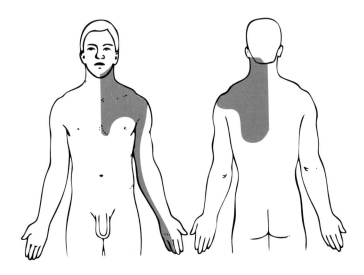

Referral Patterns from the Heart

Peripheral Arterial Disease

Peripheral arterial disease (PAD) often accompanies cardiovascular disease. The risks factors are similar to cardiovascular disease, with cigarette smoking being most directly correlated with PAD. It has been reported that individuals with PAD who are smokers exhibit a 50% increase in mortality at a 5 year follow-up.[4]

Patients with PAD often report lower extremity claudication or cramping and rest pain defined as pain on the dorsum of the foot that wakes the patient at night as a result lack of blood supply and insufficient oxygenation of the tissues. [5]

Deep Vein Thrombosis

A deep vein thrombosis (DVT) is a vascular disease which consists of venous stasis and hypercoagubility in the venous system and at times can become mobile and result in a pulmonary embolus and potentially death.[1]

The following clinical prediction rule can help a clinician identify a DVT:[6]

1. Active cancer (treatment ongoing, within previous 6 mo, or palliative) = **1 point**.
2. Paralysis, paresis, or recent plaster immobilization of the lower extremities = **1 point**.
3. Recently bedridden for >3 days or major surgery within 4 wk = **1 point**.
4. Localized tenderness along the distribution of the deep venous system. Tenderness along the deep venous system is assessed by firm palpation in the center of the posterior calf, the popliteal space, and along the area of the femoral vein in the anterior thigh and groin = **1 point**.
5. Entire lower extremity swelling = **1 point**.
6. Calf swelling > 3 cm when compared with the asymptomatic lower extremity. Measured with a tape measure 10 cm below tibial tuberosity = **1 point**.
7. Pitting edema (greater in the symptomatic lower extremity) = **1 point**.
8. Collateral superficial veins (nonvaricose) = **1 point**.
9. Alternative diagnosis as likely or greater than that of proximal DVT. More common alternative diagnoses are cellulitis, calf strain, Baker cyst, or postoperative swelling= **-2 points**.

The total score for all items is tallied and the probability of the patients having a DVT are as follows: 0=low, 1-2=moderate, and ≥3=high.[6]

Medical Screening

Gastrointestinal

Gastrointestinal (GI) symptoms can often be confused as originating from the musculoskeletal system.[7]
Further questioning of the GI system should include:[1]

1. *Have you noted discoloration of urine or blood in your stools?*
2. *Are your symptoms exacerbated after eating?*
3. *Have you vomited recently?*
4. *Have you experienced any changes in your bowel or bladder habits?*

Recently predictors of abdominal pain that are likely musculoskeletal in nature have been identified.[8] The following questions and responses from the patients exhibited a sensitivity of .67, specificity of .84, a positive likelihood ratio of 4.2, and a negative likelihood ratio of .39. The patient responds "yes" to the following 2 questions:

1. *Does coughing, sneezing, or taking a deep breath make your pain feel worse?*
2. *Do activities such as bending, sitting, lifting, twisting, or turning over in bed make your pain feel worse?*

The patient responds "no" to the following question:

1. *Has there been any change in your bowel habits since the start of your symptoms?*

If in addition to the responses to the previous questions the patient also reports "no" to the following 2 questions, then the sensitivity was .67, specificity .96, positive likelihood ratio 16.8, and negative likelihood ratio of .34.

1. *Does eating certain foods make your pain feel worse?*
2. *Has your weight changed since your symptoms started?*

The reliability of these questions ranged from moderate (kappa = .56) to very good (kappa = .88).

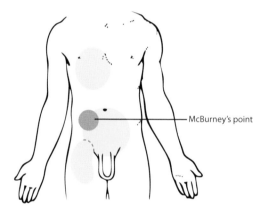

McBurney's point

Pain patterns associated with the appendix

Medical Screening

Genitourinary

The clinician should also screen for the presence of any genitourinary issues during the initial examinations. Specific questions entail:[1]

1. *Have you experienced any incontinence?*
2. *Have you noticed any blood in your urine or feces?*
3. *Have you experienced any problems with impotence?*
4. *Have you experienced any burning during urination or dysuria?*

Answers of "yes" to the aforementioned questions should lead to questioning the patient's sexual history.[9]

1. *How many sexual partners have you had?*
2. *Are the sexual partners male or female?*
3. *Was the sexual act vaginal, anal, or oral?*
4. *Was any form of protection used?*
5. *Have you experienced a past history of sexually transmitted diseases?*

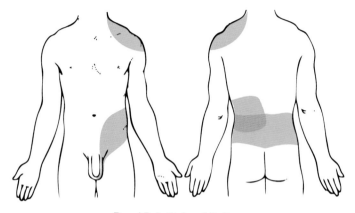

Renal Pain Referral Pattern

Endocrine

Patients with endocrine disorders are classified as having either hypo or hyperfunction and may report fluctuations in levels of fatigue, irritability, or sensitivity to temperature changes. The individuals should be queried regarding the presence of:[1,10]

1. *Polydypsia*
2. *Polyuria*
3. *The presence of an onset of confusion*
4. *Changes in hair or nail growth*
5. *Diaphoresis*
6. *Dehydration*
7. *Alterations in breathing patterns*

Pulmonary System

Screening questions directed at the pulmonary system should be performed in patients with any reports of difficulty breathing, pain with breathing, altered breathing patterns, or exhibits over the lung field on the anterior, lateral, or posterior chest wall.[1] The following questions should be asked to further ascertain involvement of the pulmonary system.[11]

1. *Do you smoke now, and did you smoke in the past? How much?*
2. *Have you experienced a cough?*
a. *If so has the cough been producing sputum? If yes, the color of the sputum and the presence of blood should be investigated.*
3. *Have you experienced any episodes of (difficult or labored breathing dyspnea) or difficulty breathing when upright (orthopnea)?*
4. *Have you experienced any episodes where you could not catch your breath?*

Medical
Screening

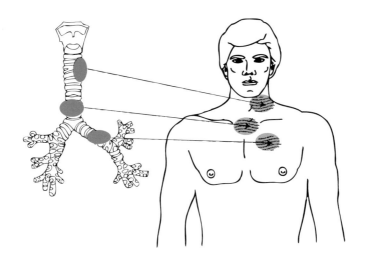

Referred pain from tracheobronchial irritation

Integumentary System

The following questions should be asked to further ascertain involvement of the integumentary system:[12]

1. *Have you recently experienced any rashes?*
2. *Have you recently noticed any enlargement or bleeding of moles?*
3. *Have you recently noticed any burning or itching of the skin?*
4. *Have you noticed any large areas of exfoliation of the skin?*
5. *Have you noticed any blistering of the skin?*

If the patient reports "yes" to any of the aforementioned questions a physical examination of the patient's skin should be performed to determine the presence of any primary skin lesions.

Medical
Screening

Primary skin lesions that may require referral include:[12]

- Macule- Circumscribed, flat change in color of skin; <1.0 cm in diameter.
- Patch- Circumscribed flat lesion; >1.0 cm in diameter
- Papule- Raise solid lesion; <0.5 cm in diameter
- Plaque- Circumscribed, raised superficial lesion with flat surface; >0.5 cm in diameter.
- Nodule- Circumscribed, raised, firm lesion; >0.5 cm in diameter.
- Wheal- Firm, raised, pink/red swelling of the skin; size and shape varies; usually itchy; lasts < 24 hours.
- Tumor- Large papule or nodule; usually > 1.0 cm in diameter.
- Pustule- Circumscribed, raised lesion containing purulent exudate that may be cloudy, white, yellow, or hemorrhagic.
- Vesicle- Circumscribed, raised lesion; filled with liquid or semi-solid material.
- Bulla- Vesicle >0.5 cm in diameter.
- Cyst- Firm, raised, encapsulated lesion; filled with liquid or semi solid material.

Neurologic Disorders

Clinicians should investigate for any signs of neurological deficits associated with either upper motor neuron or lower motor neuron involvement. Higher brain functions such as consciousness, and mental status should also be examined.

The clinician should ask the following questions:

1. *Have you been experiencing any headaches or vision changes?*
2. *Have you been experiencing any dizziness or vertigo?*
3. *Have you been experiencing any seizures or unconsciousness?*
4. *Do you ever experience the presence of any weakness or parasthesias?*

Medical Screening

Mini-Mental Examination

Clinicians can investigate the cognitive status by using two questions from the Mini-Mental Exam[13] including time orientation and the Serial Sevens Test. The clinician first performs the time orientation test by asking the patient the date including the month, day of the month, day of the week, year, and the season. The patient receives one point for each correct answer for a maximum total of five points for this question. Next the clinician asks the patients to count backwards from 100 by sevens. The patient is allowed to respond with five answers. A point is awarded for each answer that is correct for a total of five maximum points.[13] Combining the total scores for the time orientation and Serial Sevens tests yields a maximum of 10 points.

Recently Onishi and colleagues[14] demonstrated that a cut-off score of 7 for the two tests yielded a sensitivity of 98.2% and a specificity of 69.2% for identifying cognitive impairments in older adults.

Depression Screening

Depression is often not recognized in patients presenting to primary care with reports of other symptoms. Even if it is recognized that a patient presents with depression, it is likely that they won't receive an intervention to treat their depression.[15] If the patient presents with depression along with a musculoskeletal disorder, such as back pain, a multidisciplinary treatment approach could potentially maximize patient outcomes.[16]

Arroll and colleagues[17] demonstrated the utility of a two-question depression screening test in a primary care setting:

1. *During the past month have you often been bothered by feeling down, depressed, or hopeless?*
2. *During the last month have you often been bothered by little interest or pleasure in doing things?*

If the patient answered the two questions as "yes" then the sensitivity was 97% and specificity was 67%. The likelihood ratio for a positive test was 2.9 and the negative likelihood ratio was .05.

Haggman and colleagues[18] demonstrated that the above two questions were more accurate in identifying if a patient presented with depression than a physical therapist's assessment of the patient.

Medical Screening

Conclusion

The importance of developing an astute level of competence in screening for red flags should not be underestimated. Screening for red flags provides considerable guidance in the clinical decision making process relative to the best course of management.

Once a thorough screening examination has been performed and any systemic disorder ruled out with a degree of confidence, the clinician can begin to address the patient's musculoskeletal complaint directly.

Reference List

(1) Goodman CC, Snyder TEE. Differential diagnosis in physical therapy. 3rd ed. Philadelphia: W.B. Saunders Company, 2000.

(2) Sieggreen M. A contemporary approach to peripheral arterial disease. *Nurse Pract* 2006;31:14-5.

(3) Boissonnault WG. Examination in Physical Therapy Practice: Screening for Medical Disease. 2nd ed. *Philadelphia: Churchill Livingstone*, 1995.

(4) Criqui MH, Langer RD, Fronek A et al. Mortality over a period of 10 years in patients with peripheral arterial disease. *N Engl J Med* 1992;326:381-6.

(5) Sieggreen M. A contemporary approach to peripheral arterial disease. *Nurse Pract* 2006;31:14-5.

(6) Wells PS, Hirsh J, Anderson DR et al. A simple clinical model for the diagnosis of deep-vein thrombosis combined with impedance plethysmography: potential for an improvement in the diagnostic process. *J Intern Med* 1998;243:15-23.

(7) Yelland MJ. Back, chest and abdominal pain. How good are spinal signs at identifying musculoskeletal causes of back, chest or abdominal pain? *Aust Fam Physician* 2001;30:908-12.

(8) Sparkes V, Prevost AT, Hunter JO. Derivation and identification of questions that act as predictors of abdominal pain of musculoskeletal origin. *Eur J Gastroenterol Hepatol* 2003;15:1021-7.

(9) Jolley S. Taking a sexual history: the role of the nurse. *Nurs Times* 2002;98:39-41.

(10) Goodman CC. The Endocrine and Metabolic Systems. In: Goodman CC, Boissonnault WG, eds. Pathology: Implications for the Physical Therapist. Philadelphia: *W.B. Saunders*, 1998:262.

(11) Goodman CC. The Respiratory System. In: Goodman CC, Boissonnault WG, eds. Pathology: Implications for the Physical Therapist. Philadelphia: W.B. Saunders, 1998:399-455.

(12) Cole JM, Gray-Miceli D. The necessary elements of a dermatologic history and physical evaluation. *Dermatol Nurs* 2002;14:377-83.

(13) Folstein MF, Folstein SE, McHugh PR. "Mini-Mental State". A practical method for grading the cognitive state of patients for the clinician. *J Psychiatr Res* 1975;12:189-98.

(14) Onishi J, Suzuki Y, Umegaki H et al. Which two questions of Mini-Mental State Examination (MMSE) should we start from? *Arch Gerontol Geriatr.* 2006.

(15) Cohen M, Nicholas M, Blanch A. Medical assessment and managment of work related low back or neck arm pain: more questions than answers. *J Occup Health Safety Aust NZ* 2000;16:307-17.

(16) Middleton P, Pollard H. Are chronic low back pain outcomes improved with co-management of concurrent depression? *Chiropr Osteopat* 2005;13:8.

(17) Arroll B, Khin N, Kerse N. Screening for depression in primary care with two verbally asked questions: cross sectional study. *BMJ* 2003;327:1144-6.

(18) Haggman S, Maher CG, Refshauge KM. Screening for symptoms of depression by physical therapists managing low back pain. *Phys Ther* 2004;84:1157-66.

ULQ

UPPER AND LOWER QUARTER NEUROLOGICAL SCREENING

In This Chapter:

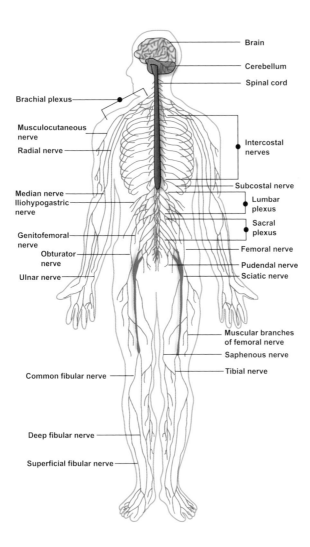

Figure of Nervous System

ULQ

Cranial Nerve Number and Function	Test
I: Olfactory Sensory from olfactory epithelium.	Assess the ability to smell common scents.
II: Optic Sensory from retina of eyes.	Assess peripheral vision by having person read an eye chart.
III: Oculomotor Motor to muscles controlling upward, downward, and medial eye movements, as well as pupil constriction.	Assess pupil constriction as a reaction to light.
IV: Trochlear Motor to muscles controlling downward and inward eye movements.	Assess the ability to move eye downward and inward by asking patient to follow your finger.

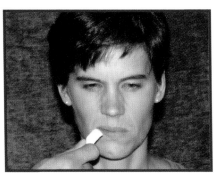

Olfactory Nerve

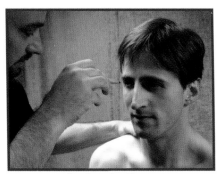

Oculomotor Nerve

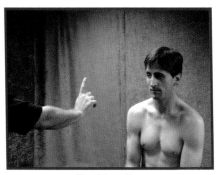

Trochlear Nerve

ULQ

Cranial Nerve Number and Function	Test
V: Trigeminal Sensory from face and motor to muscles of mastication.	Test sensation of face and cheeks as well as corneal reflex. Assess the patient's ability to clench the teeth.
VI: Abducens Motor to muscles that move eye laterally.	Assess patient's ability to move eyes away from midline by asking him to follow your finger with his eyes.
VII: Facial Motor to muscles of facial expression and sensory to anterior tongue.	Assess symmetry and smoothness of facial expressions. Test taste on anterior 2/3 of tongue.
VIII: Vestibulocochlear Hearing and balance.	Assess by rubbing fingers by each ear. Patient should hear both equally. Can also ask patient to perform balance test.

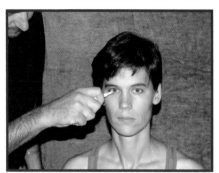

Trigeminal Nerve

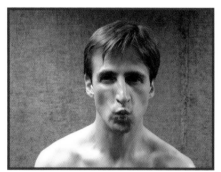

Facial Nerve

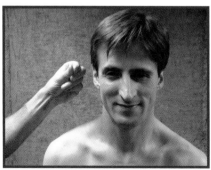

Vestibulocochlear Nerve

ULQ

Cranial Nerve Number and Function	Test
IX: Glossopharyngeal Controls gag reflex and sensory to posterior tongue.	Assess gag reflex and taste on the posterior tongue.
X: Vagus Controls muscles of pharynx, which facilitate swallowing. Provides sensory to thoracic and abdominal visceral region.	Ask patient to say "ah" and watch for elevation of soft palate.
XI: Accessory Motor to trapezius and sternocleidomastoid muscles.	Muscle testing of trapezius.
XII: Hypoglossal Motor to muscles of the tongue.	Ask patient to stick tongue straight out. Tongue will deviate toward injured side.

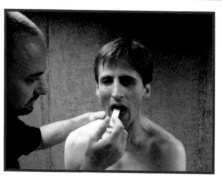

Glossopharyngeal Nerve

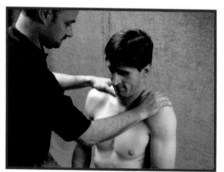

Accessory Nerve

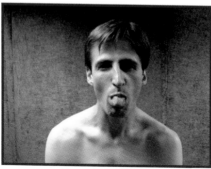

Hypoglossal Nerve

Examination of Myotomes

Strength of myotomes is assessed along with reflexes and sensation to determine the presence of nerve root involvement.

Cervical Nerve Roots

The strength of key muscles of each myotome is tested bilaterally from C1-2 through T1 to assess for the presence of cervical nerve root involvement. Manual muscle testing is performed bilaterally. Grading is either WNL (equal bilaterally) or diminished (less strength than the other side). All testing is performed with the patient seated.

Nerve Root Level, Major Muscles Innervated, and Test Procedure

---

C1 and C2:
Innervation: Muscles that flex the neck
Procedure: The examiner stabilizes the trunk with one hand and applies a posteriorly directed force through the patient's forehead while matching the resistance.

C3:
Innervation: Muscles that sidebend the neck
Procedure: The examiner stabilizes the shoulder with one hand and applies a force away from the side to be tested while the patient is instructed to match the resistance.

C4:
Innervation: Muscles that elevate the shoulders
Procedure: The patient is instructed to elevate their shoulders. The examiner applies an inferiorly directed force through the shoulders while the patient is instructed to match the resistance.

C5:
Innervation: Deltoids
Procedure: The patient is instructed to abduct their shoulders to 90 degrees. The examiner applies a force into adduction while the patient resists.

ULQ

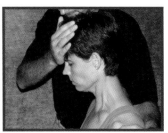

Neck Flexion

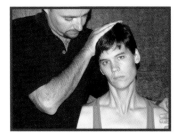

Neck Sidebending

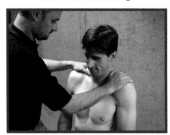

Shoulder Elevation

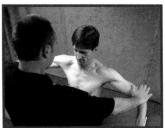

Shoulder Abduction

Nerve Root Level, Major Muscles Innervated, and Test Procedure

C6:
Innervation: Biceps and extensor carpi radialis brevis and longus
Procedure:
1. The patient's elbow is flexed to 90 degrees and the forearm supinated. The examiner applies a force into extension while the patient resists.
2. The patient's elbow is flexed to 90 degrees, forearm pronated, and wrist extended and radially deviated. The examiner applies a force into flexion and ulnar deviation while the patient resists.

C7:
Innervation: Triceps and flexor carpi radialis
Procedure:
1. The patient's elbow is flexed to 90 degrees and the examiner applies a force into elbow flexion while the patient resists.
2. The patients elbow is flexed to 90 degrees with the wrist flexed and radially deviated with forearm supinated. The examiner applies a force into wrist extension and ulnar deviation while the patient resists.

C8:
Innervation: Abductor pollicis brevis.
Procedure: The examiner places the thumb in abduction. The examiner applies a resistance through the proximal phalanx in the direction of abduction while the patient resists.

T1:
Innervation: First dorsal interossei
Procedure: The examiner separates the index and middle finger and applies a force against the lateral aspect of proximal phalanx of the index finger into adduction.

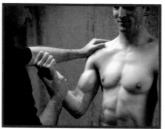

Elbow Flexion

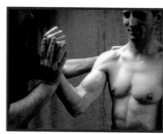

Elbow Extension

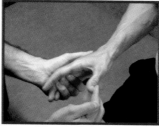

Thumb Abduction

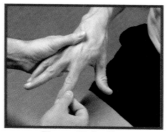

Finger Abduction

ULQ

Lumbosacral Nerve Roots

The strength of key muscles of each myotome is tested bilaterally for nerve roots from L2 through S2. Manual muscle testing is performed bilaterally. Grading is either WNL (equal bilaterally) or diminished (less strength than the other side). All testing is performed with the patient seated.

Nerve Root Level, Major Muscles Innervated, and Test Procedure

---

L2-L3:
Innervation: Hip flexors
Procedure: The patient flexes the hip to near end range and the examiner applies a force to the anterior thigh into hip extension while the patient resists.

L3-L4:
Innervation: Knee extensors
Procedure:
1. The patient extends the knee to a position slightly less than full extension. The examiner stabilizes the patient's thigh with one hand and applies pressure on the anterior distal tibia into knee flexion with the other while the patient resists.
2. Step-Up: The patient is instructed to step up onto a step stool. If the patient exhibits difficulty this could suggest involvement of the L3-L4 nerve root.

L4:
Innervation: Ankle dorsiflexors
Procedure: The patient dorsiflexes the ankle with slight inversion. The examiner stabilizes the distal tibia with one hand and the other hand applies pressure on the dorsum of the foot into plantar flexion with some eversion while the patient resists.

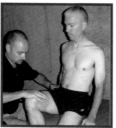

Hip Flexion

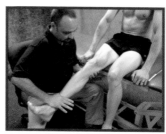

Knee Extension

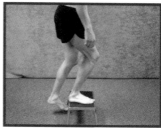

Step-Up Test

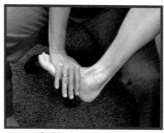

Ankle Dorsiflexion

ULQ

Lumbosacral Nerve Roots (continued)

Nerve Root Level, Major Muscles Innervated and Test Procedure

L5:
Innervation: Hallux extension
Procedure: The great toe is placed into extension. The examiner stabilizes the foot with one hand and applies pressure on the dorsum of the distal phalanx of the great toe into flexion while the patient resists.

L5-S1:
Innervation: Ankle plantar flexors
Toe-Raise: The patient is asked to rise up on the toes. Inability or difficulty to do so in relation to the opposite side may be indicative of involvement of the L5-S1 nerve root.

S1-S2:
Innervation: Ankle evertors
Procedure: The ankle is placed in full eversion and dorsiflexion. The examiner stabilizes the distal tibia with one hand and with the other hand applies pressure on the lateral aspect of the foot into plantar flexion and inversion while the patient resists.

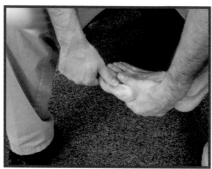

Hallux Extension

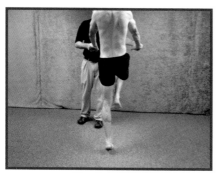

Toe-Raise Test

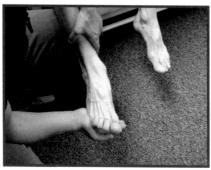

Ankle Eversion

ULQ

Sensory Examination: Segmental Nerve Root Level

Sensory testing is performed to determine the presence of nerve root or peripheral nerve involvement. Sensory examination is carried out with a pinprick (or a paper clip) in the specified anatomic areas bilaterally while the patient has the eyes closed. The patient is asked if a sharp sensation is of equal intensity on both sides, or if one side feels duller than the other, or if one side cannot be felt.

Cervical Spine

The following sensory examination (dermatomes) is assessed along with reflexes and myotomes to determine the presence of nerve root involvement. Cervical nerve root segments from C1 through T1 should be tested.

Nerve Root Level and Area of Sensory Distribution (Dermatome) Tested

C1:
Dermatomal Area: Top of head

C2:
Dermatomal Area: Posterior occipital region

C3:
Dermatomal Area: Side of neck

C4:
Dermatomal Area: Top of shoulder

C5:
Dermatomal Area: Lateral deltoid

C6:
Dermatomal Area: Tip of thumb

C7:
Dermatomal Area: Distal middle finger

C8:
Dermatomal Area: Distal fifth finger

T1:
Dermatomal Area: Medial forearm

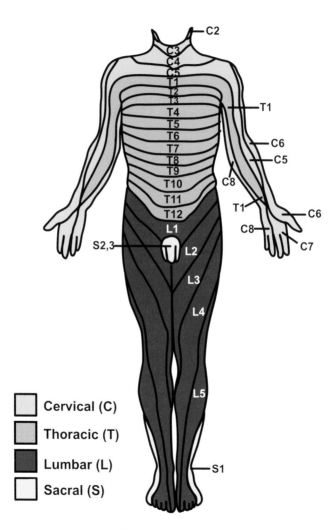

Dermatomes of the
Upper and Lower Quarter

Lumbosacral Spine

The following sensory examination (dermatomes) is assessed along with reflexes and myotomes to determine the presence of nerve root involvement. Lumbosacral nerve root segments form L1 through S4 should be tested.

Nerve Root Level and Area of Sensory Distribution (Dermatome) Tested

L1:
Dermatomal Area: inguinal region

L2:
Dermatomal Area: anterior mid-thigh

L3:
Dermatomal Area: distal anterior thigh

L4:
Dermatomal Area: medial lower leg/foot

L5:
Dermatomal Area: lateral leg/foot

S1:
Dermatomal Area: lateral side of foot

S2:
Dermatomal Area: plantar surface of foot

S3:
Dermatomal Area: groin

S4:
Dermatomal Area: perineum region, genitals

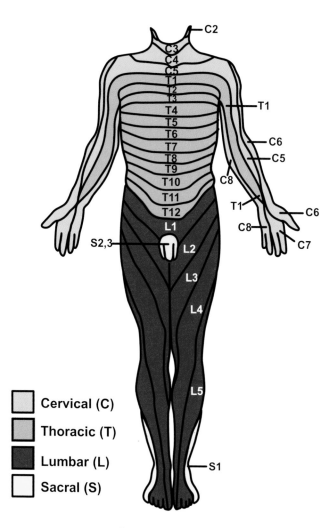

ULQ

Dermatomes of the
Upper and Lower Quarter

Sensory Examination: Peripheral Nerve Fields

Patients may demonstrate sensory deficits that do not occur in a particular dermatomal distribution. In this case the patient may exhibit a peripheral nerve lesion. Sensation can be assessed for the peripheral nerves of both the upper and lower extremities.

Upper Extremities:

The following sensory examination is used to determine the presence of a peripheral nerve lesion in the upper extremities. Sensory examination is carried out with a pinprick (or a paper clip) in the specified anatomic areas bilaterally while the patient has the eyes closed. The patient is asked if a sharp sensation is of equal intensity on both sides, or if one side feels duller than the other, or if one side cannot be felt.

Peripheral Nerve and Area of Sensory Distribution Tested

Musculocutaneous Nerve:
Sensory Distribution: Radial border of forearm

Axillary Nerve:
Sensory Distribution: Lateral deltoid

Radial Nerve:
Sensory Distribution: Dorsum of radial side of wrist

Median Nerve:
Sensory Distribution: Palmar surface of first 3 digits and radial half of digit 4

Ulnar Nerve:
Sensory Distribution: Palmar surface of digit 5 and ulnar half of digit 4

ULQ

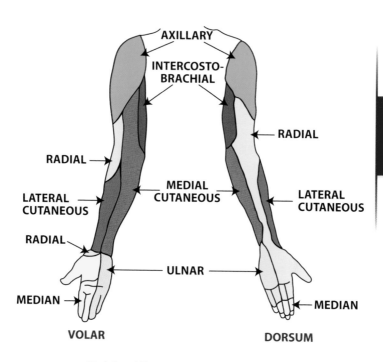

Peripheral Nerve Fields of Upper Extremity

Lower Extremities:

The following sensory examination is used to determine the presence of a peripheral nerve lesion in the lower extremities. Sensory examination is carried out with a pinprick (or a paper clip) in the specified anatomic areas bilaterally while the patient has their eyes closed. The patient is asked if a sharp sensation is of equal intensity on both sides, or if one side feels duller than the other, or if one side cannot be felt.

Peripheral Nerve and Area of Sensory Distribution Tested

Lateral Femoral Cutaneous Nerve:
Sensory Distribution: Lateral thigh

Obturator Nerve:
Sensory Distribution: Medial thigh

Femoral Nerve:
Sensory Distribution: Medial aspect of leg from the middle thigh distal to the medial malleolus

Sciatic Nerve:
Sensory Distribution: Posterior thigh, posterior distal calf, dorsum and lateral border of the foot

Superficial Peroneal Nerve:
Sensory Distribution: Dorsum of the foot

Deep Peroneal Nerve:
Sensory Distribution: Dorsum of the foot between the 1st and 2nd toe

Sural Nerve:
Sensory Distribution: Lateral border of foot

Tibial Nerve:
Sensory Distribution: Plantar surface of the foot

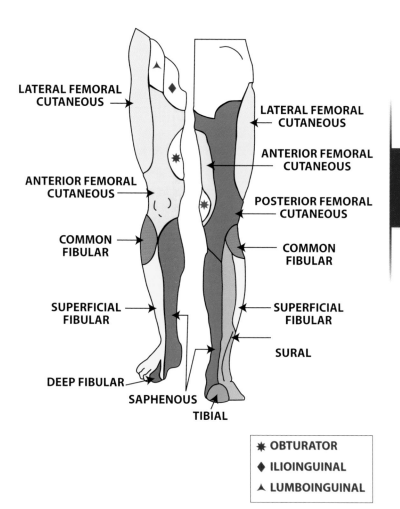

LATERAL FEMORAL CUTANEOUS

LATERAL FEMORAL CUTANEOUS

ANTERIOR FEMORAL CUTANEOUS

ANTERIOR FEMORAL CUTANEOUS

POSTERIOR FEMORAL CUTANEOUS

COMMON FIBULAR

COMMON FIBULAR

SUPERFICIAL FIBULAR

SUPERFICIAL FIBULAR

SURAL

DEEP FIBULAR

SAPHENOUS

TIBIAL

ULQ

✳ OBTURATOR
◆ ILIOINGUINAL
▲ LUMBOINGUINAL

Peripheral Nerve Fields of Lower Extremity

Lower Motor Neuron Reflexes

The following muscle stretch reflexes are tested bilaterally with the patient seated. Each reflex is graded as absent/diminished, WNL, or hyperactive. Reflexes found to be diminished or absent can be correlated with the dermatome and myotome assessments to determine the presence of nerve root pathology. Those that are hyperactive may indicate upper motor neuron pathology.

Cervical Reflexes

Reflex, Corresponding Cervical Nerve Root Level, and Procedure

Biceps Brachii (C5 nerve root):

Procedure: The patient's arm is placed in about 45° of flexion with the muscle relaxed. The examiner strikes the tendon in the cubital fossa, just proximal to the bicep insertion. The thumb may be placed over the tendon to insure proper technique. The examiner observes for elbow flexion.

Brachioradialis (C6 nerve root):

Procedure: The patient's arm is placed in about 45° of flexion with the muscle relaxed. The examiner strikes the tendon at the distal aspect of the radius with the flat edge of the reflex hammer. The examiner observes for elbow flexion.

Triceps (C7 nerve root):

Procedure: The examiner supports the patient's arm and strikes the triceps tendon just proximal to the olecranon. The examiner observes for elbow extension.

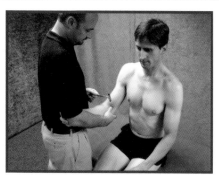

Biceps Reflex

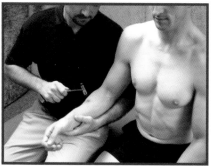

Brachioradialis Reflex

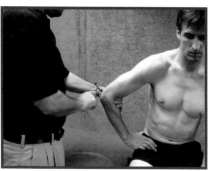

Triceps Reflex

Lumbar Reflexes

All of the following reflex testing will be performed with the patient seated.

Quadriceps (L4):

Procedure: The examiner taps the patellar tendon and observes for knee extension.

Achilles (S1)

Procedure: The examiner grasps the patient's foot and places it into slight dorsiflexion. The examiner then taps the Achilles tendon and observes and feels for ankle plantar flexion.

ULQ

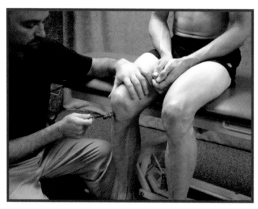

Quadriceps Reflex

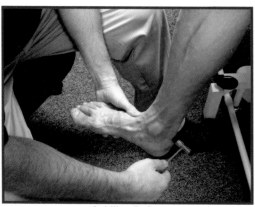

Achilles Reflex

Upper Motor Neuron Reflexes

The following reflexes are tested to determine the presence of a central nervous system disorder.

Reflex, Test Procedure, and Criteria for Positive Findings

Hoffman's Reflex:

Procedure: The patient is seated with the head in a neutral position. The examiner flicks the distal phalanx of the middle finger. The test is considered positive if there is flexion of the interphalangeal joint of the thumb, with or without flexion of the index finger proximal or distal interphalangeal joints.

Babinski Sign:

Procedure: The patient is supine. The examiner strokes the plantar surface of the foot with a fingernail or instrument from posterior lateral toward the ball of the foot . The test is considered positive if the great toe extends and the other toes fan out.

Clonus:

Procedure: The patient is seated or supine. The examiner rapidly dorsiflexes the ankle. Test is considered positive if the quick stretch results in reflexive twitching of the plantarflexors.

Romberg Test:

Procedure: the patient is standing with feet close together. The patient is then instructed to close the eyes. The test is considered positive if the amount the patient sways is increased with eyes closed or if the patient loses balance.

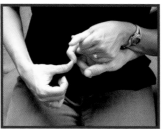

Hoffman's Reflex

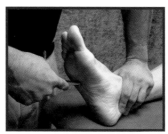

Babinski Sign

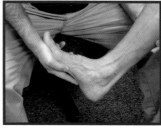

Testing for Clonus

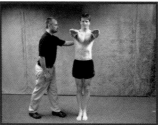

Romberg Test

ULQ

CERVICOTHORACIC SPINE EXAMINATION

In This Chapter:

1. Historical Examination
2. Observation, Functional Tests, & Palpation Active Range of Motion, Passive Range of Motion, & Overpressures
   a. Flexion
   b. Extension
   c. Sidebending
   d. Rotation
   e. Combined Movement
   3. Resisted Muscle Tests
   a. Deep Neck Flexor Endurance

4. **Assessments of Accessory Movements**
   a. Posterior-Anterior Segmental Mobility

5. **Special Tests**
   a. Spurling's Test
   b. Cervical Rotation Lateral Flexion (CRLF) Test
   c. Sharp Purser Test
   d. Distraction Test
   e. Upper Limb Tension Test
   f. Test Item Cluster for Cervical Radiculopathy

Region Specific Historical Examination:

In addition to the historical examination presented in Chapter three, patient should be asked specific questions related to the cervical and thoracic spine and surrounding regions:

1. *Do you get symptoms into the legs or low back with neck movements?*
   — If "yes" a detailed neurological examination should be performed.

2. *Have you experienced any bilateral upper extremity symptoms or occasional loss of balance or lack of coordination in the lower extremities?*
   — If "yes" a detailed neurological examination should be performed.

3. *The following questions have some utility in identifying patients with cervical radiculopathy.*[7]

Question	+ LR (yes)	- LR (no)
Do neck movements improve your symptoms?	2.2	.50
Where is the pain most bothersome? Answer - Shoulder and scapula.	2.3	

CT Spine

Radiographs and Cervical Spine Trauma

The Canadian C-Spine (cervical-spine) Rule (CCR) is a decision rule to guide the use of cervical-spine radiography in patients with trauma. The purpose of the rule is to identify the need for radiography in alert and stable patients that have suffered a cervical spine injury.[1,2]

Diagnostic Accuracy[1]

Target Condition: A clinically important cervical spine injury, including any fracture, dislocation, or ligamentous instability demonstrated on imaging.

Sensitivity = 99.4 %

Specificity = 45.1 %

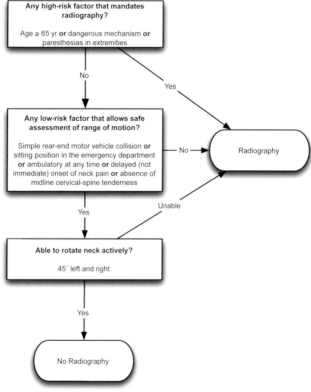

Canadian C-Spine Rule

Observation

Watch the patient walk and observe any abnormal gait mechanics, particularly signs of upper motor neuron involvement such as ataxia or synergy patterns.

With the patient sitting, the examiner observes for any asymmetries in any of the soft tissues or bony landmarks of the cervical and thoracic spine and the upper extremities. The examiner should observe the patient from the anterior, posterior, and lateral views.

Functional Tests

The patient should demonstrate any functional movement or activity that reproduces symptoms. These functional movements often include one or more of the following activities:

— looking up
— transferring from sit to stand
— lifting one or both arms overhead

CT Spine

Palpation

The examiner palpates the thorax starting superficial and progressing to deeper structures. The examiner palpates for the presence of any temperature changes, moisture, soft tissue or lymph node swelling, and tissue texture abnormalities.

Symmetry of bony landmarks is observed including the rib angles, the region overlying the transverse processes, and the upper ribs anteriorly.

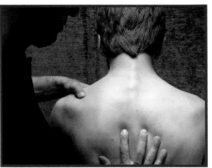

Transverse Processes

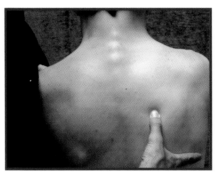

Rib Angle

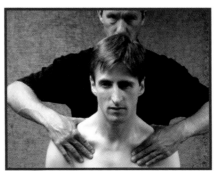

Upper Rib Cage

Active Range of Motion (AROM), Passive Range of Motion (PROM), & Overpressures:

With the patient sitting, the examiner asks the patient to perform the following motions while assessing the quality and quantity of motion and change in symptoms, particularly if symptoms move distally from the spine ("peripheralization"). After performing active range of motion, the examiner passively moves the cervical spine through maximal range of motion (as tolerated by the patient), applies overpressure, and assesses range of motion, pain reproduction, and end-feel. ROM can be quantified with a standard goniometer or gravity/bubble inclinometer.

Flexion

The patient is asked to look down towards the floor. The quality of the motion is noted and the distance from the chin to the sternum is noted. Overpressure can be applied at the end range of motion while the examiner stabilizes the upper thorax.

Extension

The patient is asked to look up towards the ceiling. The quality of the motion is noted. Overpressure can be applied at the end range of motion while the examiner stabilizes the upper thorax.

Sidebending

The patient is asked to drop the ear toward the shoulder.. The quality of the motion is noted and the distance from the ear to the shoulder is noted. Overpressure can be applied at the end range of motion while the examiner stabilizes the opposite shoulder and upper thorax.

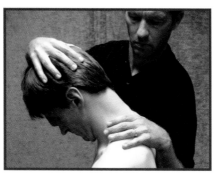

Flexion

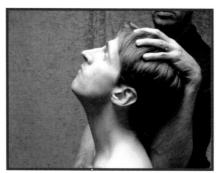

Extension

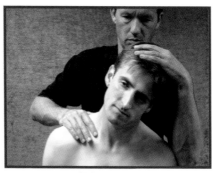

Sidebending

Active Range of Motion (AROM), Passive Range of Motion (PROM), & Overpressures:

Observe Eyes
Sitting - The patient is asked to look over the shoulder. The examiner notes the presence of dizziness, lightheadedness, nystagmus, impaired sensation to the face, blurred vision, or other signs or symptoms consistent with compromise to the vertebrobasilar complex. It is repeated to the other direction.

Rotation
Sitting - The patient is asked to look over the shoulder. The quality of the motion is noted. Overpressure can be applied at the end range of motion.

Combined Extension, Sidebending, Rotation (Quadrant)
Sitting - The patient is asked to look up and over the shoulder. The quality of the motion is noted. Overpressure can be applied at the end range of motion while the examiner stabilizes the shoulder.

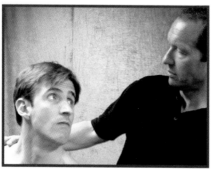

Observe Eyes

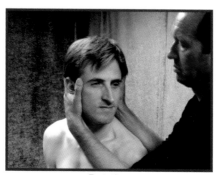

Rotation

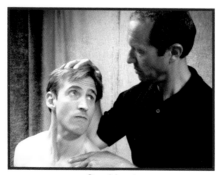

Combined

Active Range of Motion of the Ribcage:

With the patient supine the examiner palpates directly over the ribs anteriorly and asks the patient to make a full inspiratory and expiratory effort. Typically the ribcage is divided into thirds, and assessment is made of the respiratory excursion for the upper ribs, the middle ribs, and the lower ribs. The examiner observes which group of ribs stops moving first during either inhalation or exhalation.

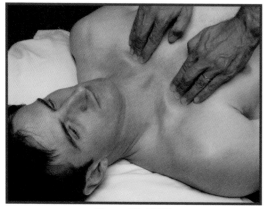

Upper Rib ROM

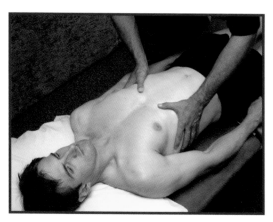

Lower Rib ROM

Resisted Muscle Tests:

Resisted tests are performed isometrically and are performed to assess strength and symptom response. The following selected resisted tests can be performed when examining the cervical-thoracic region.

Deep Neck Flexor Endurance

Craniocervical flexion endurance is designed to assess the deep neck flexor muscles and the longus capitus and colli. The patient is supine and is asked to flex the knees to 90° and place the soles of the feet flat on the table. The patient is asked to tuck the chin in and lift the head off of the examiners finger tips. The examiner observes for substitution of the sternocleidomastoid muscle. The time to fatigue is measured in seconds.

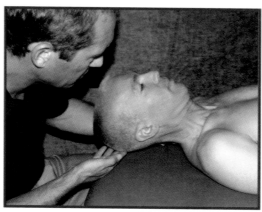

Deep Neck Flexor Endurance

Assessments of Accessory Movements

The examiner investigates accessory movement of the individual cervical spine segments. With all tests, pain responses are recorded and mobility judgments are established as hypermobile, normal, or hypomobile.

Posteroanterior Mobility

Purpose:
To test for segmental movement and pain response.

Description:
The patient is prone. The examiner contacts the spinous process with the thumbs. The lateral neck musculature is gently pulled posteriorly with the fingers. The examiner should be directly over the contact area keeping elbows extended.. The examiner uses the upper trunk to impart a posterior to anterior force in a progressive and oscillatory fashion over the spinous process. Repeat for remaining cervical segments.

Positive Test:
The test result is considered to be positive if the patient reports reproduction of pain. The mobility of the segment is judged to be normal, hypermobile, or hypomobile.

Diagnostic Accuracy:
Pain during segmental testing was associated with reports of neck pain.[3]
Sensitivity = .82   - LR = .23
Specificity = .79   + LR = 3.9

Reliability:
Kappa = .14 – .37 (pain)[4]
ICC = .42 – .79 (pain)[5]

CT
Spine

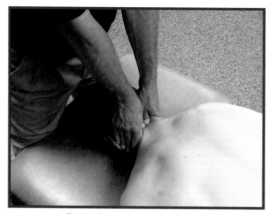

Posterior to anterior mobility

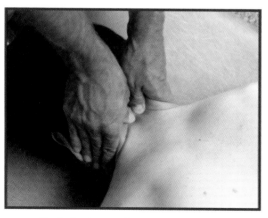

Posterior to anterior mobility- Close Up

Assessments of Accessory Movements

The examiner investigates accessory movement of the individual cervical spine segments. With all tests, pain responses are recorded and mobility judgments are established as hypermobile, normal, or hypomobile.

Segmental Mobility

Purpose:
To test for segmental movement and pain response.

Description:
The patient is supine.

C2-C7- The examiner contacts the articular pillars (posterior facet region) with the proximal phalanx of the 2nd digit. The head and neck are flexed up to the segment and a lateral side flexion glide from right to left and left to right is performed at each level. It is repeated with the neck slightly extended to the level of interest.

C1-C2- The examiner contacts C1 with the proximal phalanx of the 2nd digit just inferior to the occiput. The head and neck are flexed and the examiner slowly turns the upper cervical spine and head to the right and then the left.

Occipital-Atlanto- The examiner supports the occiput in the hands. The patient's neck is rotated approximately 30 degrees to the right. The examiner slowly nods the head up and down. This is repeated rotating to the left.

Positive Test:
The test result is considered to be positive if the patient reports reproduction of pain. The mobility of the segment is judged to be normal, hypermobile, or hypomobile.

Diagnostic Accuracy:
Unknown

Reliability:[6]
Kappa = .03 – .63 (mobility)
ICC = .22 – .80 (pain)

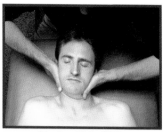

Flexion Side Glide

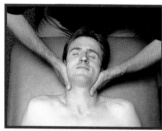

Extension Side Glide

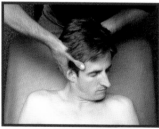

Atlanto Axial Mobility

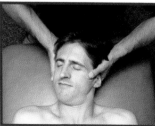

Occipital Atlanto Mobility

CT
Spine

Special Tests:

Spurling's Test

Purpose:
To test for the presence or absence of cervical radiculopathy.

Description:
The patient is seated. The examiner sidebends the neck towards the affected side and applies approximately 7 kg of compression force.

Positive Test:
The test is considered positive if symptoms are reproduced.

Diagnostic Accuracy:[7]
Reference standard cervical radiculopathy as diagnosed by needle electromyography and nerve conduction studies.
Sensitivity = .50   - LR = .58
Specificity = .86   + LR = 3.5

Reliability:
Kappa = .60[7]

CT
Spine

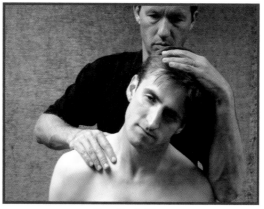

Spurling's Test

Cervical Rotation Lateral Flexion (CRLF) Test

Purpose:
To test for the presence of 1st rib hypomobility in patient's with brachialgia.[8]

Description:
The test is performed with the patient in sitting. The cervical spine is passively and maximally rotated away from the side being tested. While maintaining this position, the spine is gently flexed as far as possible moving the ear toward the chest.

Positive Test:
A test is considered positive when the lateral flexion movement is blocked.

Diagnostic Accuracy:[9]
The reference standard is presence of rib hypomobility on cineradiography in subjects with brachialgia.
Kappa = .84

Reliability:
Kappa = 1.0

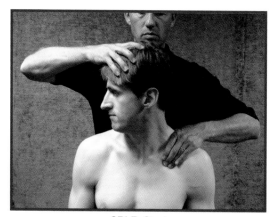

CRLF- Start

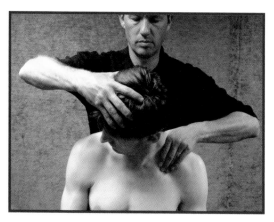

CRLF- End

Sharp-Purser Test

Purpose:
To test for the presence of upper cervical spine instability.

Description:
The patient is seated in a semiflexed position. The examiner places the palm of one hand on the patient's forehead and index finger of the other hand on the spinous process of the axis. Posterior pressure is applied through the forehead.

Positive Test:
The test is considered positive if a sliding motion of the head posterior occurs. This is often accompanied by a reduction in symptoms.

Diagnostic Accuracy:[10]
Reference standard is an atlanto-dens interval greater than 3 mm on full flexion and extension lateral radiographs.

Sensitivity = .69   - LR = .32
Specificity = .96   + LR = 17.3

Reliability:
Unknown

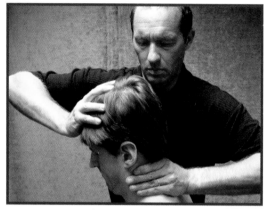

Sharp-Purser Test

Cervical Distraction Test

Purpose:
To test for the presence of cervical radiculopathy.

Description:
The patient is supine and the examiner is seated. The examiner grasps under the chin and occiput while slightly flexing the patient's neck and applies a distraction force of ~ 14 lbs.

Positive Test:
The test is considered to positive if the patients symptoms are reduced.

Diagnostic Accuracy:[7]
Reference standard cervical radiculopathy as diagnosed by needle electromyography and nerve conduction studies.
Sensitivity = .44   - LR = .62
Specificity = .90   + LR = 4.4

Reliability:
Inter-examiner Kappa = .88

CT Spine

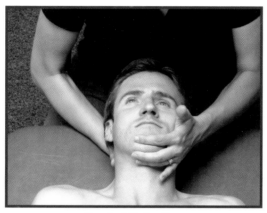

Cervical Distraction

Upper Limb Tension Test A (ULLT)

Purpose:
To test for the presence of cervical radiculopathy.

Description:
The patient is supine. The examiner performs the following movement sequence:
- Scapular depression
- Shoulder abduction
- Forearm supination, wrist and finger extension
- Shoulder lateral elevation
- Elbow extension
- Contralateral/ipsilateral cervical side bending

Positive Test:
The test is positive if one or more of the following occurs:
- Symptoms reproduced
- Side to side difference in elbow extension greater than 10 degrees
- Contralateral cervical side bending increases symptoms, or ipsilateral side bending decreases symptoms

Diagnostic Accuracy:[7]
Reference standard cervical radiculopathy as diagnosed by needle electromyography and nerve conduction studies.

Sensitivity = .97   - LR = .12
Specificity = .86   + LR = 3.5

Reliability:
Inter-examiner Kappa = .76[7]

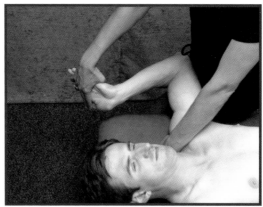

ULTT- Start

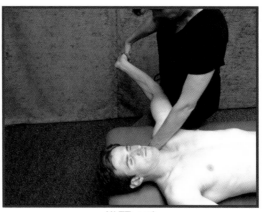

ULTT- end

CT
Spine

Test Item Cluster for the Diagnosis of Cervical Radiculopathy

Purpose:
To determine the likelihood that a patient has a cervical radiculopathy.

Description:
The following test item cluster (TIC) can be performed entirely from the physical exam without any additional lab or imaging tests.

Criterion Definition of Positive:
- + Upper limb tension test A (ULTT-A)
- + Spurling's test
- + Distraction test
- Cervical rotation less than 60 degrees to the ipsilateral side

Diagnostic Accuracy:[7]
3 positive tests from the TIC
+ LR = 6.1

4 positive tests from the TIC
+ LR = 30.3

Test Item Cluster for Patients with Mechanical Neck Pain Likely to Benefit from Thoracic Spine Manipulation

Purpose:
To identify patients with neck pain who are likely to experience early success with thoracic spine thrust manipulation.[11]

Description:
The following test item clusters (TIC) can be performed entirely in the history and physical exam, without any additional lab or imaging tests.

Criterion Definition of Positive:
- Symptoms less than 30 days
- No symptoms distal to the shoulder
- Looking up does not aggravate symptoms
- FABQ Physical Activity Score less than 12
- Diminished upper thoracic spine kyphosis
- Cervical extension ROM less than 30°

Diagnostic Accuracy:[11]
Reference standard success was a 5 point or greater level of improvement on the Global Rating of Change (GRC).

3 positive tests from the TIC
+ LR = 5.5

4 positive tests from the TIC
+ LR = 12.0

5 positive tests from the TIC
+ LR = Infinite

All 6 positive tests from the TIC
+LR = Infinite

Reference List

(1) Stiell IG, Clement CM, McKnight RD, et al. The Canadian C-Spine rule versus the NEXUS low-risk criteria in patients with trauma. *N Engl J Med* 2003:2510-2518.

(2) Stiell IG, Wells GA, Vandemheen KL, et al. The Canadian C-spine rule for radiography in alert and stable trauma patients. *JAMA* 2001;286:1841-1848.

(3) Sandmark H, Nisell R. Validity of five common manual neck pain producing tests. *Scand J Rehabil Med* 1995;27:131-136.

(4) van Suijlekom H, deVet H, van den Berg S, Weber W. Interobserver reliability in physical examination of the cervical spine in patients with headache. *Headache* 2000;40:581-586.

(5) Bertilison B, Grunnesjo M, Strender L. Reliability of clinical tests in teh assessment of patients with neck/shoulder problems. Impact of history. *Spine*. 2003;28:2222-2231.

(6) Pool J, Hoving J, Henrica C, et al. The interexaminer reproducibity of physical examination of the cervical spine. *J Manipulative Physiol Ther* 2004;27:84-90.

(7) Wainner RS, Fritz JM, Irrgang JJ, et al. Reliability and diagnostic accuracy of the clinical examination and patient self-report measures for cervical radiculopathy. *Spine* 2003;28:52-62.

(8) Lindgren K-A, Leino E, Hakola M, Hamberg J. Cervical spine rotation and lateral flexion combined motion in the examination of the thoracic outlet. *Arch Phys Med Rehabil* 1990;71:343-344.

(9) Lindgren K-A, Leino E, Manninen H. Cineradiography of the hypomobile first rib. *Arch Phys Med Rehabil* 1989;70:408-409.

(10) Uitvlugt G, Indenbaum S. Clinical assessment of atlantoaxial instability using the Sharp-Purser test. *Arthritis Rheum* 1988;31:918-922.

(11) Cleland J, Childs J, Fritz J, et al. Development of a clinical prediction rule for guiding treatment of a subgroup of patients with neck pain: use of thoracic spine manipulation, exercise, and patient education *Phys Ther* 2007;87:9-23.

Shoulder

SHOULDER EXAMINATION

In This Chapter:

Region Specific Historical Examination:

The patient should be asked specific questions related to the shoulder and surrounding regions.

1. *Do your symptoms change (better or worse) with any movements of the neck?*

   If the patient answers "yes" this indicates the cervical spine should be evaluated in detail.

2. *Does your arm ever slip out or feel unstable?*

   If the patient answers "yes" this could be suggestive of instability.

3. *Does your pain change with overhead activities?*

   If patient answers "yes" this could indicate possible subacromial impingement syndrome.[1]

4. *Do you have difficulty moving your arm?*

   If the patient answers "yes" you should follow-up by asking if they have difficulty moving the arm because of pain or it just won't move. The latter may be indicative of rotator cuff tear.[2]

5. *Does your arm ever feel heavy after performing activities?*

   If patient answers "yes" this may be indicative of vascular compromise.

Shoulder

Observation and Palpation:

This portion of the examination should be performed with the patient either standing or seated.

Observation

With the patient seated and standing the examiner observes for any asymmetries in any of the soft tissues or bony landmarks.

Position of the cervical, thoracic, and lumbar spine as well as the resting position of the elbow, forearm, wrist, and hand should be observed.

The examiner should observe the patient from the anterior, posterior, and lateral views.

Palpation

The examiner palpates the upper quadrant starting superficially and progressing to deeper structures. The examiner palpates for the presence of any temperature changes, moisture, swelling, and tissue texture abnormalities.

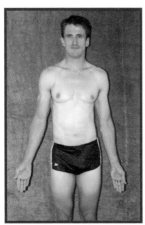

Anterior View

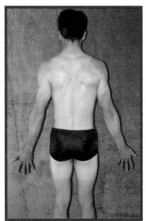

Posterior View

Shoulder

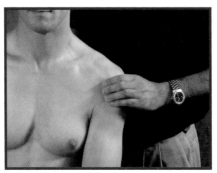

Palpation

Active Range of Motion, Passive Range of Motion and Overpressure:

With the patient seated or standing the examiner asks the patient to perform the following motions to assess the quality and quantity of motion and change in symptoms. Active range of motion can be quantified with a standard goniometer or inclinometer. Following active range of motion testing the therapist moves the joint through maximal range of motion (as tolerated by the patient), applies overpressure, and assesses range of motion, pain reproduction, and end-feel.

Flexion and Extension
The patient is asked to raise the arms into flexion, then extension in the sagittal plane.

Abduction and Adduction
The patient is asked abduct the arms in the frontal plane and then return them to the side.

Internal Rotation and External Rotation
The patient is asked to perform internal rotation and external rotation with the shoulder in a neutral position as well as in 90 degrees of flexion.

Horizontal Abduction and Adduction
The patient is asked to abduct the arms to 90 degrees and move the arms first posteriorly then anteriorly in the transverse plane.

Hand Behind Back
The patient is asked to bring the arm behind the back and reach up the back as high as possible. The vertebral level reached by the tip of the longest finger is recorded. This allows for the assessment of the following combined motions, internal rotation, extension and adduction.

Hand Behind Head
The patient is asked to bring the arm behind their head and reach down as far as possible. The vertebral level reached by the tip of the longest finger is recorded. This allows for the assessment of the following combined motions: external rotation, flexion, and adduction.

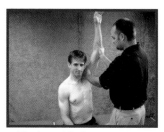

Flexion with Overpressure

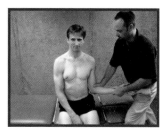

External Rotation with
Overpressure

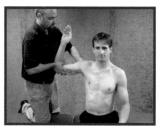

Horizontal Abduction with
Overpressure

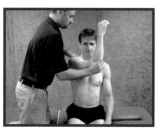

Horizontal Adduction with
Overpressure

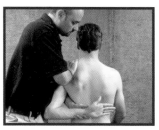

Hand Behind Back with
Overpressure

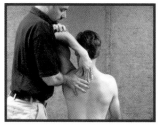

Hand Behind Head with
Overpressure

Resisted Muscle Tests:

Resisted tests are performed isometrically and are performed to assess symptom response and strength of the muscles. The following list provides selected resisted tests that should be performed when examining the shoulder region.

Shoulder Flexion

The examiner asks the patient to flex the arm to 90 degrees while the examiner stabilizes the shoulder with one hand. The patient is then asked to resist an inferiorly directed force produced by the examiner through the patient's forearm.

Shoulder Abduction

The examiner asks the patient to abduct the shoulder while the examiner stabilizes the shoulder with one hand. The patient is then asked to resist an inferiorly directed force produced by the examiner through the patient's forearm.

Shoulder Internal and External Rotation

The patient's arm is resting in neutral and the examiner flexes the elbow to 90 degrees while stabilizing the elbow with one hand. The patient is asked to resist against a laterally directed force produced by the examiner's other hand.

The patient's arm is resting in neutral and the examiner flexes the elbow to 90 degrees while stabilizing the elbow with one hand. The patient is asked to resist against a medially directed force produced by the examiner's other hand.

Shoulder

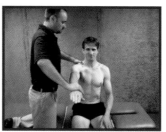

Resisted Flexion

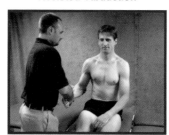

Resisted Abduction

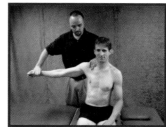

Resisted Internal Rotation

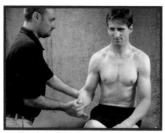

Resisted External Rotation

Assessments of Accessory Movements

The examiner investigates accessory movement of the glenohumeral, acromioclavicular, sternoclavicular, and scapulothoracic joint with the patient either supine or prone.

Techniques Performed in Supine:

Inferior Glide of Humerus

With the patient's shoulder stabilized on the table, the examiner guides the patient's arm into approximately 90 degrees of abduction with one hand. When this position is obtained, the examiner applies an inferior force at the proximal humerus and assesses the amount of mobility and symptomatic response.

Posterior Glide of Humerus

With the patient's the shoulder stabilized by the table the examiner guides the patient's arm into approximately 90 degrees of abduction with one hand. When this position is obtained, the examiner applies a posterior force at the proximal humerus and assesses the amount of mobility and symptomatic response.

Anterior/Posterior Glide of Acromioclavicular Joint

The examiner grips the distal clavicle with the index finger on the superior/posterior surface and the thumb on the anterior surface with their thumb. The examiner then glides the clavicle in an anterior and posterior direction while assessing mobility and symptoms response.

The examiner places the web space of theihand between the thenar and hypothenar eminence on the anterior aspect of the proximal clavicle and applies a posteriorly directed force. The examiner assesses mobility and symptoms.

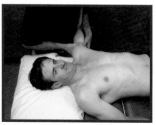

Inferior Glide of Humerus

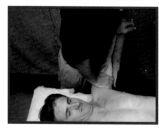

Posterior Glide of Humerus

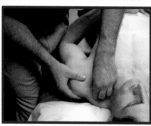

**Anterior/Posterior Glide of
Acromioclavicular Joint**

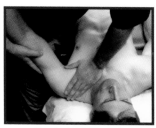

**Posterior Glide of
Sternoclavicular Joint**

Special Tests:

Active Compression Test

Purpose:
To test for the presence of an acromioclavicular lesion or a labral tear.

Description:
The patient is standing and instructed to place the shoulder in a position of 90 degrees of flexion and 10 degrees of adduction. The patient's arm is internally rotated so that the thumb is pointing down. The patient is instructed to resist an inferiorly directed force applied by the examiner first with the thumb down and then with the thumb up.

Positive Test:

1. **Acromioclavicular lesions**
   The test is considered positive if the patient reports pain localized to the acromioclavicular joint when resistance is applied with the thumb pointing down and reduced or eliminated pain when resistance is applied with the forearm supinated.

2. **Labral tears**
   The test is considered positive if the patient reports painful clicking in the glenohumeral joint occuring when resistance is applied with the thumb pointing down and reduced or eliminated pain when resistance was applied with the forearm supinated.

Diagnostic Accuracy:

1. **Acromioclavicular lesions**
   Sensitivity = .41 - 1.0   - LR =.00 - .62[3, 4]
   Specificity = .95 - .97   + LR = 8.2 - 33.3[3, 4]

2. **Labral tears**
   Sensitivity = .63 - 1.0   - LR = .00 - . 51[4, 5]
   Specificity = .73 -.98   + LR = 2.3 - 50.0[4, 5]

Reliability:
Not reported

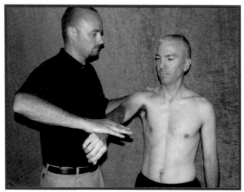

Active Compression Start Position

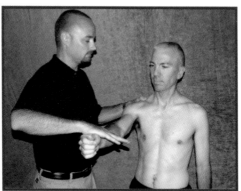

Active Compression End Position

Test Item Cluster for the Identification of Subacromial Impingement Syndrome

Purpose:
To test the presence of subacromial impingement syndrome.

Description:
The following 3 tests are performed with the patient standing: the Hawkins-Kennedy Impingement Sgn, the painful arc sign, and the infraspinatus muscle test.

Hawkins-Kennedy Impingement Sign:
The examiner places the patient's shoulder in 90 degrees of shoulder flexion with the elbow flexed to 90 and then internally rotates the arm. The test is considered to be positive if the patient experiences pain with internal rotation.

The Painful Arc Sign:
The patient is instructed to fully elevate the arm in the scapular plane and then slowly reverse the motion. This test is considered to be positive if the patient experiences pain between 60 and 120 degrees of elevation.

Infraspinatus Muscle Test:
With the arm resting in neutral, the patient is instructed to flex the elbow to 90 degrees and resist against a medially directed force. The test is considered positive if the patient exhibits pain or weakness when resistance is applied. This test is also considered to be positive if the patient's arm is externally rotated passively but falls into internal rotation when it is released by the examiner.

* If all three tests are found to be positive then the + LR is 10.56 and if all 3 are negative the - LR is .17.[6]
* If two of the three tests are positive than the +LR is 5.03[6]

Reliability:
Not reported

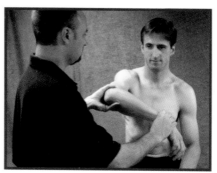

Hawkins-Kennedy Test

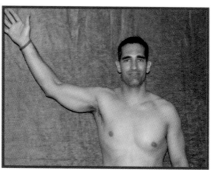

Painful Arc Sign

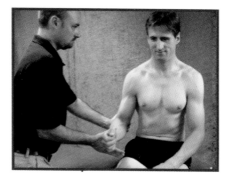

Apprehension Test

Purpose:
To test the integrity of the anterior glenohumeral joint capsule and assess for glenohumeral joint instability.

Description:
The patient is in the supine position. The examiner flexes the patient's elbow to 90 degrees and abducts the patient's shoulder to 90 degrees, maintaining neutral rotation. The examiner then slowly externally rotates the shoulder to 90 degrees while monitoring the patient.

Positive Test:
Test is considered positive if the patient exhibits signs of apprehension as the examiner brings the shoulder into external rotation.

Diagnostic Accuracy:
Sensitivity = .53   - LR = .47[7]
Specificity = .99   + LR = 53[7]

Reliability:
Kappa = .47[8]

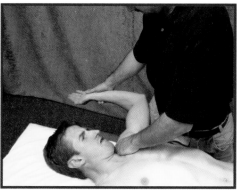

Apprehension Test

Biceps Load Test II

Purpose:
To test for the presence of a superior glenohumeral labral tear.

Description:
The patient is supine and the examiner grasps the patient's wrist with one hand and the elbow with the other. The examiner then places the patient's shoulder in a position of 120 degrees abduction, maximal external rotation, 90 degrees of elbow flexion and forearm supination. In this position the patient is asked to perform elbow flexion against resistance.

Positive Test:
If the patient reports an increase in symptoms during the resisted contraction, the test is considered positive.

Diagnostic Accuracy:
Sensitivity= .90[9]   - LR=.10[9]
Specificity= .97[9]   + LR=30[9]

Reliability:
Kappa=.82

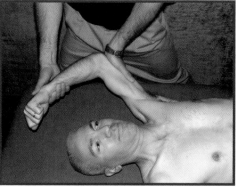

Bicep Load Test II

Shoulder

Test Item Cluster for the Identification of a Full-Thickness Rotator Cuff Tear

Purpose:
To test the presence of a full-thickness rotator cuff tear.

Description :
The following 3 tests are performed with the patient standing; the drop-arm sign, the painful arc sign, and the infraspinatus muscle test.

The Drop-Arm Sign:
The patient is asked to actively elevate the arm in the scapular plane and then slowly reverse the motion. The test is considered to be positive if the patient experiences pain or the arm drops suddenly.

The Painful Arc Sign:
The patient is instructed to fully elevate the arm in the scapular plane and then slowly return it to their side. This test is considered to be positive if the patient experiences pain or a painful catching between 60 and 120 degrees.

Infraspinatus Muscle Test:
With the arm resting in neutral, the patient is instructed to flex the elbow to 90 degrees and resist against a medially directed force. The test is considered positive if the patient exhibits pain or weakness when resistance is applied. This test is also considered to be positive if the patient's arm is externally rotated passively but falls into internal rotation when it is released by the examiner.

* If all three tests are found to be positive then the +LR is 15.6 and if all 3 are negative the –LR is .16.[6]
* If all 3 test are positive and the patient is greater than 60 years of age the +LR is 28.0[6]
* If two of the three tests are positive than the +LR is 3.6[6]

Reliability:
Not reported

Reference List

(1)   Michener LA, Walsworth MK, Burnet EN. Effectiveness of rehabilitation for patients with subacromial impingment syndrome: A systematic review. *J Hand Ther* 2004;17(2):152-64.

(2)   Litaker D, Pioro M, El BH, Brems J. Returning to the bedside: using the history and physical examination to identify rotator cuff tears. *J Am Geriatr Soc* 2000 December;48(12):1633-7.

(3)   Chronopoulos E, Kim TK, Parh HB, Ashenbrenner D, McFarland EG. Diagnostic value of physical tests for isolated chronic acromioclavicular leasions. *Am J Sports Med* 2004;32(3):655-60.

(4)   O'Brien SJ, Pangnani MJ, Fealey S, Mcglynn SR, Wilson JB. The active compression test: A new and effective test for diagnosing labral tears and acromioclavicular joint abnormality. *Am J Sports Med* 1998;26(5):610-3.

(5)   Guanche CA, Jones DC. Clinical testing for tears of the glenoid labrum. *Arthroscopy* 2003 May;19(5):517-23.

(6)   Park HB, Yokota A, Gill HS, El RG, McFarland EG. Diagnostic accuracy of clinical tests for the different degrees of subacromial impingement syndrome. *J Bone Joint Surg Am* 2005 July;87(7):1446-55.

(7)   Lo IK, Nonweiler B, Woolfrey M, Litchfield R, Kirkley A. An evaluation of the apprehension, relocation, and surprise tests for anterior shoulder instability. *Am J Sports Med* 2004 March;32(2):301-7.

(8)   Tzannes A, Paxinos A, Callanan M, Murrell GA. An assessment of the interexaminer reliability of tests for shoulder instability. *J Shoulder Elbow Surg* 2004 January;13(1):18-23.

(9)   Kim SH, Ha KI, Ahn JH, Kim SH, Choi HJ. Biceps load test II: A clinical test for SLAP lesions of the shoulder. *Arthroscopy* 2001 February;17(2):160-4.

Shoulder

ELBOW EXAMINATION

In this Chapter

1. **Historical Examination**
2. **Observation and Palpation**
3. **Active Range of Motion, Passive Range of Motion, and Overpressure**
    a. Flexion and Extension
    b. Supination and Pronation
4. **Resisted Muscle Tests**
    a. Elbow Flexion
    b. Elbow Extension
    c. Forearm Supination
    d. Forearm Pronation
5. **Assessment of Accessory Movements**
    a. Proximal Radioulnar Joint
    b. Distal Radioulnar Joint
    c. Humeroulnar Distraction
    d. Humeroradial Distraction
6. **Special Tests**
    a. Ulnar Nerve Compression Test
    b. Elbow Extension Test
    c. Varus and Valgus Stress Test
    d. Moving Valgus Stress Test
    e. Tests for Lateral Epicondylalgia

Region Specific Historical Examination:

The patient should be asked specific questions related to the elbow and surrounding regions.

1. *Do your symptoms change (better or worse) with any movements of the neck or shoulder?*

    If the patients answers "yes" this indicates the cervical spine and shoulder should be evaluated in detail.

    a. *Do you elbow ever slip out or feel unstable?*

    If the patient answers "yes" this could be suggestive of instability.

    b. *Does the pain change with gripping activities?*

    If patient answers "yes" this could indicate possible lateral or medial epicondylalgia.[1, 2]

    c. *Do you ever experience numbness or tingling in the hand?*

    If the patient answers "yes" this may indicate possible pronator or cubitual tunnel syndrome.[3]

    d. *Was the elbow hyperextended during the time of injury?*

    If patient answers "yes" this may indicate fracture of ligamentous / capsular damage.[4]

    e. *Do you relate the symptoms to a throwing activity?*

    If patient answers "yes" this may indicate medial instability.[9]

Elbow & Forearm

Observation and Palpation:

This portion of the examination should be performed with the patient either standing or seated.

Observation

With the patient seated and standing the examiner observes for any asymmetries or deformities in any of the soft tissues or bony landmarks.

Position of the cervical and thoracic spine as well as the resting position of the shoulder, elbow, forearm, wrist, and hand should be observed. The examiner observes for any valgus or varus deformities of the elbow.

The examiner should observe the patient from the anterior, posterior, and lateral views.

Palpation

The examiner palpates the elbow, forearm, and surrounding soft tissue and bony structures starting superficially and progressing to deeper structures. The examiner palpates for the presence of any temperature changes, moisture, swelling, and tissue texture abnormalities.

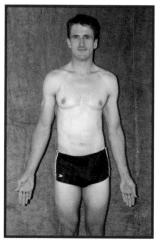

Anterior

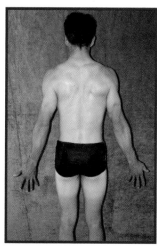

Posterior

Elbow & Forearm

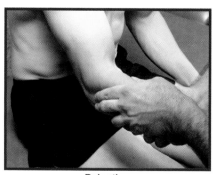

Palpation

Active Range of Motion, Passive Range of Motion, and Overpressures:

With the patient seated or standing the examiner asks the patient to perform the following motions while assessing the quality and quantity of motion and change in symptoms. Active range of motion can be quantified with a standard goniometer or inclinometer. The interrater and intrarater reliability of obtaining measurements during active range of motion, where available, can be found in the table below. Following active range of motion testing, the therapist moves the joint through maximal range of motion (as tolerated by the patient), applies overpressure, and assesses range of motion, pain reproduction, and end-feel.

Elbow Flexion:

The patient is asked to bend the elbow as far as actively possible. If no symptoms are elicited the examiner applies over pressure while assessing quality of motion, symptom response, and end feel.

Intrarater reliability: .55-.97[5-7]
Interrater reliability: .55-.96[5-7]

Elbow Extension:

The patient is asked to actively extend the elbow as far as possible. If no symptoms are elicited the examiner applies overpressure while assessing quality of motion, symptom response, and end feel.

Intrarater reliability: .45-.99[5-7]
Interrater reliability: .58-.96[5-7]

Supination and Pronation:

The patient is asked to maintain 90 degrees of elbow flexion and to supinate the forearm forearm actively as far as possible. If no symptoms are elicited the examiner applies overpressure while assessing quality of motion, symptom response, and end-feel. The procedure is then repeated in the direction of pronation.

Supination:
Intrarater reliability: .94-.99[6,8,9]
Interrater reliability: .90-.96[6,8,9]

Pronation:
Intrarater reliability: .86-.98[6,8,9]
Interrater reliability: .83-.95[6,8,9]

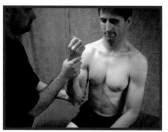

Flexion with Overpressure

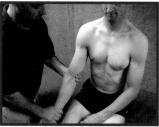

Extension with Overpressure

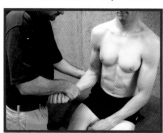

Supination with Overpressure

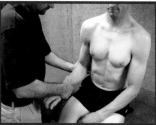

Pronation with Overpressure

Elbow &
Forearm

Resisted Muscle Tests:

Resisted muscle tests are performed isometrically and are performed to assess symptom response and strength of the muscles. The following list provides selected resisted tests that should be performed when examining the elbow region.

Elbow Flexion

The patient is seated. The examiner asks the patient to flex the elbow to 90 degrees while the examiner stabilizes the shoulder with one hand. The patient is then asked to resist an inferiorly directed force produced by the examiner through the patient's forearm.

Elbow Extension

The patient is seated. The examiner asks the patient to flex the elbow to 100 degrees while the examiner stabilizes the shoulder with one hand. The patient is then asked to resist a superiorly directed force produced by the examiner through the patient's forearm.

Forearm Supination

The patient is seated and is asked to flex the elbow to 90 degrees with the forearm in neutral (thumb pointing up). The examiner grasps the patient's distal forearm with one hand and stabilizes the elbow with the other. The patient is instructed to resist a force applied by the examiner in the direction of forearm pronation.

Forearm Pronation

The patient's is seated and is asked to flex the elbow to 90 degrees with the forearm in neutral (thumb pointing up). The examiner grasps the patient's distal forearm with one hand and stabilizes the elbow with the other. The patient is instructed to resist a force applied by the examiner in the direction of forearm supination.

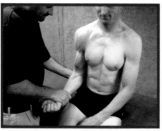

Elbow Flexion

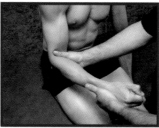

Elbow Extension

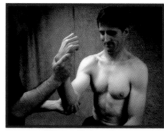

Forearm Supination

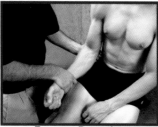

Forearm Pronation

Elbow &
Forearm

Assessment of Accessory Movements

The examiner investigates accessory movement of the humeroulnar, humeroradial, and proximal/distal radioulnar joints.

Techniques Performed Supine:

Proximal Radioulnar Joint

With the patient supine and the elbow resting on the table, the examiner slightly supinates the forearm. The examiner stabilizes the proximal ulna with one hand and firmly grasps the radial head with the other. The examiner then volarly and dorsally glides the radial head and assesses the mobility and symptom response.

Distal Radioulnar Joint

With the patient supine and the elbow resting on the table the examiner supinates the forearm. The examiner stabilizes the distal ulna with one hand and firmly grasps the distal radius with the other. The examiner then volarly and dorsally glides the distal radius and assess the mobility and symptom response.

Humeroulnar Distraction

With the patient's humerus stabilized on the table, the examiner flexes the patient's elbow to approximately 60 degrees and places both hands over the proximal ulna with fingers interlocked. The examiner then applies a distraction force and assesses the mobility and symptom response.

Humeroradial Distraction

The examiner stabilizes the patient's humerus against the table with one hand, grasps the distal radius with the other hand, and flexes the elbow to approximately 45 degrees. When this position is obtained the examiner performs a long axis distraction through the humeroradial joint and assesses the mobility and symptom response.

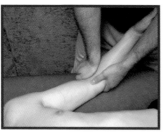

Proximal Radioulnar Joint

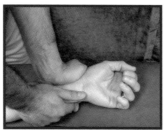

Distal Radioulnar Joint

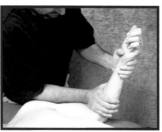

Humeroulnar Distraction

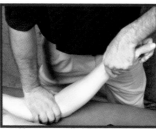

Humeroradial Distraction

Elbow &
Forearm

Special Tests:

Ulnar Nerve Compression Test

Purpose:
To test for the presence of cubital tunnel syndrome.

Description:
The patient is standing and instructed by the examiner to passively flex the elbow approximately 20 degrees. The examiner then places a firm pressure on the ulnar nerve just proximal to the cubital tunnel and maintains the pressure for 60 seconds.

Positive Test:
The test is considered positive if the patient reports numbness and/or tingling in an ulnar nerve distribution.

Diagnostic Accuracy:
Sensitivity = .89   - LR = .11[10]
Specificity = .98   + LR = 44.5[10]

Reliability:
Not reported

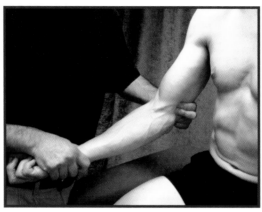

Ulnar Nerve Compression Test

Elbow &
Forearm

Elbow Extension Test

Purpose:
To test the presence of either a bony fracture or elbow joint effusion.

Description:
The patient is asked to extend the elbow as far as possible while either in a supine or standing position. The examiner makes an assessment to whether or not full extension can be achieved.

Positive Test:
The test is considered positive if the patient is unable to fully extend the elbow.

Diagnostic Accuracy:
Sensitivity = .91   - LR = .04[11]
Specificity = .70   + LR = 3.1[11]

Reliability:
Not reported

Elbow &
Forearm

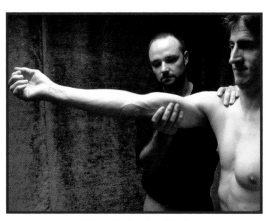

Elbow Extension Test

Varus and Valgus Stress Test

Purpose:
To test for the presence of a medial or lateral collateral ligament tear of the elbow.

Description:
Varus Stress Test:

The patient is standing. The examiner places the patient's elbow in approximately 20 degrees of flexion while palpating the lateral joint line. The examiner applies a varus force to the elbow.

Positive Test:
The test is considered positive if the patient experiences pain or excessive laxity is noted compared to the contralateral side.

Valgus Stress Test:

The patient is standing. The examiner places the patient's elbow in approximately 20 degrees of flexion while palpating the medial joint line. The examiner applies a valgus force to the elbow.

Positive Test:
The test is considered positive if the patient experiences pain or excessive laxity is noted compared to the contralateral side.

Diagnostic Accuracy:
Not reported for either test.

Reliability:
Not reported for either test.

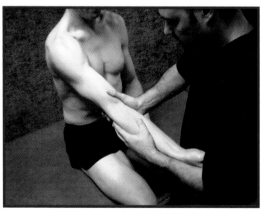

Varus Stress Test

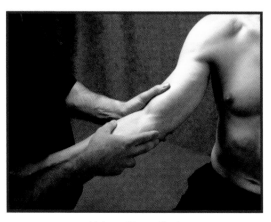

Valgus Stress Test

Moving Valgus Stress Test

Purpose:
To test for the presence of a medial collateral ligament tear of the elbow.

Description:
The patient is standing and is asked to abduct the shoulder to 90 degrees. The examiner grasps the distal forearm with one hand and stabilizes the elbow with the other. The examiner then maximally flexes the elbow and places a valgus torque to the elbow while simultaneously externally rotating the shoulder. When the shoulder reaches the end range of external rotation the examiner quickly extends the elbow to approximately 30 degrees.

Positive Test:
To be considered a positive test the two following criteria must be identified: 1. The patient experiences pain at the medial elbow, and 2. The maximal amount of pain must be experienced between 120 and 70 degrees of elbow flexion.

Diagnostic Accuracy:
Sensitivity = 1.0   - LR = 0.0[12]
Specificity = .75   + LR = 4.0[12]

Reliability:
Not reported

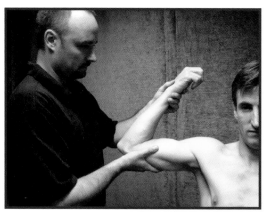

Moving Valgus Stress Test Start Position

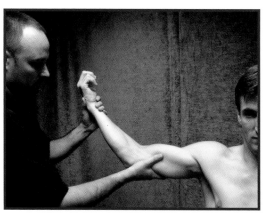

Moving Valgus Stress Test End Position

Elbow &
Forearm

Tests for Lateral Epicondylalgia

Purpose

To test the presence of lateral epicondylalgia.

Description:

While the diagnostic utility of the following tests is unknown they are typically used to identify the presence of lateral epicondylalgia: (1) pain during palpation of the lateral epicondyle, (2) pain with resisted wrist extension, or (3) pain with resisted middle finger extension.[13-15]

Pain during palpation of the lateral epicondyle:

With the patient standing or seated the examiner palpates the lateral epicondyle. A test is considered positive if the palpation reproduces the patient's symptoms.

Pain with resisted wrist extension:

With the patient seated and the forearm on the table, the patient is asked to extend the wrist. The examiner uses one hand to stabilize the forearm and the other to contact the dorsum of the hand. The patient is asked to resist the examiners force, which is applied in the direction of wrist flexion. This test is considered positive if the patient experiences pain while performing the resisted contraction.

Pain with resisted middle finger extension:

With the patient seated and the forearm on the table, the patient is asked to extend the 3rd finger. The examiner uses one hand to stabilize the forearm and the other to contact the extended 3rd finger. The patient is asked to resist the examiner's force, which is applied in the direction of finger flexion. This test is considered positive if the patient experiences pain while performing the resisted contraction.

Diagnostic Accuracy:

Not reported

Reliability:

Not reported

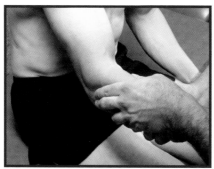

Palpation of Lateral Epicondyle

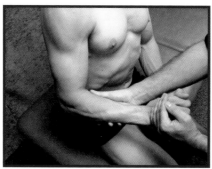

Resisted Wrist Extension

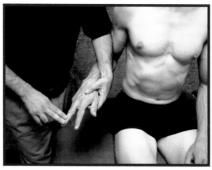

Resisted Middle Finger Extension

Elbow &
Forearm

Reference List

(1) Vicenzino B, Wright A. Lateral epicondylalgia I: epidemiology, pathophysiology, aetiology and natural history. *Phys Ther Rev* 1996;1:23-34.

(2) Wright A, Vicenzino B. Lateral epicondylalgia II: Therapeutic management. *Phys Ther* 1997;2:39-48.

(3) Kingery WS, Park KS, Wu PB, Date ES. Electromyographic motor Tinel's sign in ulnar mononeuropathies at the elbow. *Am J Phys Med Rehabil* 1995 November;74(6):419-26.

(4) O'Driscoll SW. Elbow instability. *Hand Clin* 1994 August;10(3):405-15.

(5) Rothstein J, Miller P, Roettger R. Goniometric reliability in a clinical setting. Elbow and knee measurements. *Phys Ther* 1983;63(10):1611-5.

(6) Armstrong AD, MacDermid JC, Chinchalkar S, Stevens RS, King JW. Reliability of range-of-motion measurement in the elbow. *J Elbow Shoulder Surg* 1998;7:573-80.

(7) Boone D, Azen S, Lin J, Baron C, et al. Reliability of goniometric measurements. *Phys Ther* 1978;58(11):1355-60.

(8) Gajdosik RL. Comparison and reliability of three goniometric methods for measuring forearm supination and pronation. *Percept Mot Skills* 2001 October;93(2):353-5.

(9) Karagiannopoulos C, Sitler M, Michlovitz S. Reliability of 2 functional goniometric methods for measuring forearm pronation and supination active range of motion. *J Orthop Sports Phys Ther* 2003 September;33(9):523-31.

(10) Novak CB, Lee GW, Mackinnon SE, Lay L. Provocative testing for cubital tunnel syndrome. *J Hand Surg [Am]* 1994 September;19(5):817-20.

(11) Hawksworth CR, Freeland P. Inability to fully extend the injured elbow: an indicator of significant injury. *Arch Emerg Med* 1991 December;8(4):253-6.

(12) O'Driscoll SW, Lawton RL, Smith AM. The "moving valgus stress test" for medial collateral ligament tears of the elbow. *Am J Sports Med* 2005 February;33(2):231-9.

(13) Pienimaki T, Tarvainen T, Siira P, Malmivaara A, Vanharanta H. Associations between pain, grip strength, and manual tests in the treatment evaluation of chronic tennis elbow. *Clin J Pain* 2002 May;18(3):164-70.

(14) Pienimaki TT, Siira PT, Vanharanta H. Chronic medial and lateral epicondylitis: a comparison of pain, disability, and function. *Arch Phys Med Rehabil* 2002 March;83(3):317-21.
(15) Waugh EJ, Jaglal SB, Davis AM, Tomlinson G, Verrier MC. Factors associated with prognosis of lateral epicondylitis after 8 weeks of physical therapy. *Arch Phys Med Rehabil* 2004 February;85(2):308-18.

Elbow &
Forearm

WRIST AND HAND EXAMINATION

In This Chapter:

1. **Historical Examination**
2. **Observation and Palpation**
3. **Active Range of Motion, Passive Range of Motion, and Overpressure**
   a. Wrist Flexion
   b. Wrist Extension
   c. Radial Deviation
   d. Ulnar Deviation
   e. Finger Flexion/Extension
   f. Thumb Abduction/Adduction
4. **Resisted Muscle Tests**
   a. Wrist Flexion
   b. Wrist Extension
   c. Radial Deviation
   d. Ulnar Deviation
   e. Finger Flexion
   f. Finger Extension
5. **Assessment of Accessory Movements**
   a. Radiocarpal Dorsal Glide
   b. Radiocarpal Volar Glide
   c. Radiocarpal Radial/Ulnar Glide
   d. Dorsal/Volar Glide of MCP, PIP, and DIP Joints
6. **Special Tests**
   a. Axial Loading of the Thumb
   b. Scaphoid Shift Test
   c. Finkelstein Test
7. **Carpal Compression Test**
8. **Clinical Prediction Rule for Diagnosing Carpal Tunnel Syndrome**

Region-Specific Historical Examination:

The patient should be asked specific questions related to the hand and surrounding regions.

1. *Do your symptoms change (better or worse) with any movements of the neck, shoulder, or elbow?*
   If the patient answers "yes" this indicates the cervical spine, shoulder or elbow should be examined in detail.

2. *Do you have a traumatic injury and pain when loading the wrist?*
   If the patient answers "yes" this could be suggestive of a scaphoid fracture or carpal instability.[1, 2]

3. *Do you ever experience numbness or tingling in the hand?*
   If the patient reports "yes" this could indicate possible carpal tunnel syndrome or compression of the ulnar nerve at the tunnel of Guyon.[3, 4]

4. *Does shaking the hands decreases the symptoms?*
   If patient answers "yes" this may indicate carpal tunnel syndrome[5]

5. *Do you have difficulty extending the finger specifically in the morning?*
   If patient answers "yes" this may indicate possible DeQuervain's syndrome.[6]

6. *Do you have increased pain with gripping activities requiring radial deviation of the wrist?*
   If patient answers "yes" this may indicate possible DeQuervain's syndrome.[2]

Hand & Wrist

Observation and Palpation:

This portion of the examination should be performed with the patient seated.

Observation

With the patient seated the examiner observes for any asymmetries in any of the soft tissues or bony landmarks.

Position of the cervical and thoracic spine as well as the resting position of the shoulder, elbow, forearm, wrist, and hand should be observed. The examiner observes the normal resting position of the hand and fingers. In addition, the examiner observes for any deformities of the fingers (and finger nails) that may be suggestive of a systematic disorder.

The examiner should observe the patient from the anterior, posterior, and lateral views.

Palpation

The examiner palpates the hand and surrounding soft tissue and bony structures starting superficially and progressing to deeper structures. The examiner palpates for the presence of any temperature changes, moisture, swelling, and tissue texture abnormalities.

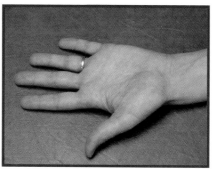

Palmar Surface

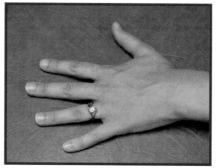

Dorsal Surface

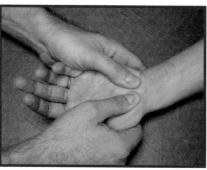

Palpation

Hand & Wrist

Active Range of Motion, Passive Range of Motion, and Overpressure:

With the patient seated the examiner asks the patient to perform the following motions to assess the quality and quantity of motion and change in symptoms. Active range of motion can be quantified with a standard goniometer or inclinometer. The interrater and intrarater reliability of obtaining measurements during active range of motion can be found in the table below. Following active range of motion testing the therapist moves the joint through maximal range of motion (as tolerated by the patient), applies overpressure, and assesses range of motion, pain reproduction, and end-feel.

Wrist Flexion

The patient is asked to flex the wrist as far as actively possible. If no symptoms are elicited the examiner applies overpressure while assessing quality of motion, symptom response, and end-feel.

Intrarater reliability: .96[7]
Interrater reliability: .90[7]

Wrist Extension

The patient is asked to actively extend the wrist as far as possible. If no symptoms are elicited the examiner applies overpressure while assessing quality of motion, symptom response, and end feel.

Intrarater reliability: .96[7]
Interrater reliability: .85[7]

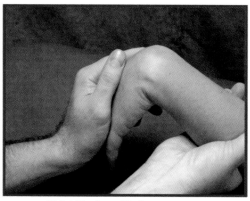

Wrist Flexion with Overpressure

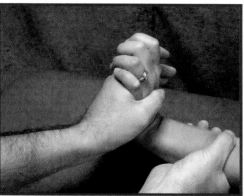

Wrist Extension with Overpressure

Hand &
Wrist

Active Range of Motion, Passive Range of Motion and Overpressure: Continued

Radial Deviation

The patient is asked to actively radially deviate the wrist as far as possible. If no symptoms are elicited the examiner applies overpressure while assessing quality of motion, symptom response, and end feel.

Intrarater reliability: .90[7]
Interrater reliability: .86[7]

Ulnar Deviation

The patient is asked to actively ulnarly deviate the wrist as far as possible. If no symptoms are elicited the examiner applies overpressure while assessing quality of motion, symptom response, and end-feel.

Intrarater reliability: .76-.92[7, 8]
Interrater reliability: .72-.78[7, 8]

Finger Flexion/Extension

The patient flexes or extends the fingers at each respective joint (MCPs, PIPs and DIPs). If no symptoms are elicited the examiner applies overpressure while assessing quality of motion, symptom response, and end-feel. Flexion and extension of the first digit occur in the frontal plane.

Intrarater reliability for flexion/extension of IPs: .97-.98[9]
Interrater reliability for flexion/extension of IPs: .97[9]

Thumb Abduction and Adduction

The patient abducts and adducts the thumb. If no symptoms are elicited the examiner applies overpressure while assessing quality of motion, symptom response, and end-feel. Abduction and adduction of the first digit occur in the sagittal plane.

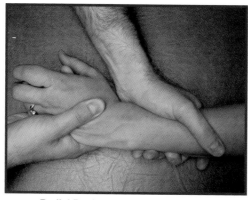

Radial Deviation with Overpressure

Hand &
Wrist

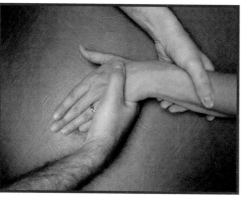

Ulnar Deviation with Overpressure

Resisted Muscle Tests:

Resisted muscle tests are performed isometrically and are performed to assess symptom response and strength of the muscles. The following list provides selected resisted tests that should be performed when examining the hand region.

Wrist Flexion

The patient is seated. The examiner asks the patient to flex the wrist while the examiner stabilizes the forearm with one hand. The patient is then asked to resist a force applied by the examiner in the direction of wrist extension.

Wrist Extension

The patient is seated. The examiner asks the patient to extend the wrist while the examiner stabilizes the forearm with one hand. The patient is then asked to resist a force applied by the examiner in the direction of wrist flexion.

Radial Deviation

The patient is seated. The examiner asks the patient to radially deviate the wrist while the examiner stabilizes the forearm with one hand. The patient is then asked to resist a force applied by the examiner in the direction of ulnar deviation.

Ulnar Deviation

The patient is seated. The examiner asks the patient to ulnarly deviate the wrist while the examiner stabilizes the forearm with one hand. The patient is then asked to resist a force applied by the examiner in the direction of radial deviation.

Finger Flexion

The patient is seated. The examiner asks the patient to individually flex digits 2-4 while the examiner stabilizes the wrist and hand with one hand. The patient is then asked to resist a force applied by the examiner in the direction of finger extension. The same technique can be used for the first digit in isolation.

Finger Extension

The patient is seated. The examiner asks the patient to extend digits 2-4 while the examiner stabilizes the hand and wrist with one hand. The patient is then asked to resist a force applied by the examiner in the direction of finger flexion. The same technique can be used for the first digit in isolation.

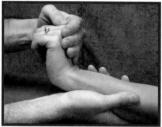

Resisted Wrist Extension

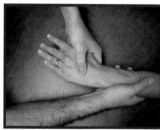

Resisted Wrist Radial Deviation

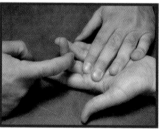

Resisted Finger Flexion

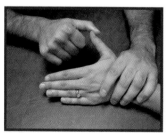

Resisted Thumb Extension

Hand &
Wrist

Assessment of Accessory Movements

The examiner investigates accessory movement of the radiocarpal, MCP, PIP, and DIP joints with the patient seated.

Radiocarpal Dorsal Glide

With the patient seated and the forearm resting on the table, the examiner places the forearm in supination. The examiner stabilizes the forearm with one hand and firmly grasps the carpals with the other. The examiner then dorsally glides the carpals and assesses the amount of mobility and symptom response.

Radiocarpal Volar Glide

With the patient seated and the forearm resting on the table, the examiner places the forearm in pronation. The examiner stabilizes the forearm with one hand and firmly grasps the carpals with the other. The examiner then volarly glides the carpals and assesses the amount of mobility and symptom response.

Radiocarpal Radial/Ulnar Glide

With the patient seated and the forearm resting on the table, the examiner places the forearm in neutral supination/pronation (thumb pointing up). The examiner stabilizes the forearm with one hand, firmly grasping the carpals with the other. The examiner then alternately radially and ulnarly glides the carpals and assesses the amount of mobility and symptom response.

Dorsal/Volar Glide of MCPs, IPs, and DIPs

With the patient seated the examiner identifies the respective joint to be tested. The examiner then stabilizes the proximal bone (as close to the joint as possible) and with the other hand grasps the distal bone (as close to the joint as possible) and then glides the distal segment in either a dorsal or volar direction. For example, to assess the glide at the 2nd MCP joint the examiner stabilizes the metacarpal with one hand while using the other to glide the proximal phalanx.

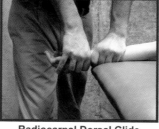

Radiocarpal Dorsal Glide

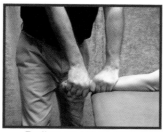

Radiocarpal Volar Glide

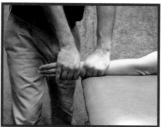

Radiocarpal Ulnar Glide

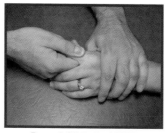

Dorsal Glide 2nd MCP

Hand &
Wrist

Special Tests:

Axial Loading of the Thumb

Purpose:
To test for the presence of a scaphoid fracture.

Description:
The patient is seated and the forearm is supported on the table. The examiner passively abducts and extends the thumb at the MCP joint. The examiner then applies a compressive load through the first CMC joint by applying an axial load through the metacarpal bone.

Positive Test:
The test is considered positive if the patient reports pain when compression is applied.

Diagnostic Accuracy:
Sensitivity = .89   - LR = .02[10]
Specificity = .98   + LR = 49[10]

Reliability:
Not reported

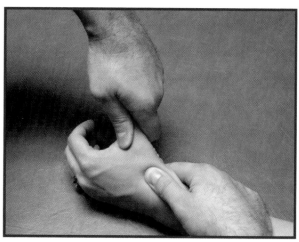

Axial Loading of the Thumb

Scaphoid Shift Test

Purpose:
To test for the presence of scaphoid instability.

Description:
The patient is seated with the forearm pronated and stabilized on the table. The examiner grasps the radial side of the patient's wrist with one hand with the thumb over the scaphoid. The examiner's other hand grasps the hand at the level of the metacarpals. The examiner maintains firm compression over the scaphoid while passively taking the patient into ulnar deviation and slight extension, then slowly into radial deviation and slight flexion. In the final position the examiner releases the compression on the scaphoid.

Positive Test:
The test is considered positive if a "thunk" is produced or the patient's symptoms are reproduced when compression of the scaphoid is released.

Diagnostic Accuracy:
Sensitivity = .69   - LR = .47[11]
Specificity = .66   + LR = 2.0[11]

Reliability:
Not reported

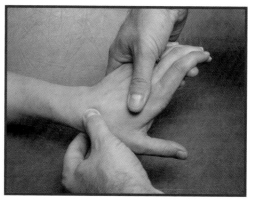

Scaphoid Shift Test: Ulnar Deviation and Slight Extension

Hand & Wrist

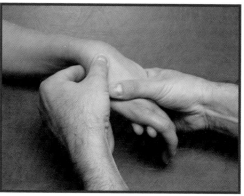

Scaphoid Shift Test: Radial Deviation and Slight Flexion

Finkelstein Test

Purpose:
To test for the presence of tenosynovitis of the abductor pollicis longus and extensor pollicis brevis tendons in the first dorsal tunnel of the wrist (DeQuervain's disease).

Description:
The patient is standing or seated and is instructed to make a fist with the thumb between the palm and fingers. The examiner then stabilizes the forearm with one hand and passively ulnarly deviates the wrist.[4]

Positive Test:
The test is considered positive if pain over the radial styloid process is reproduced with ulnar deviation.[4]

Diagnostic Accuracy:
Not reported

Reliability:
Not reported

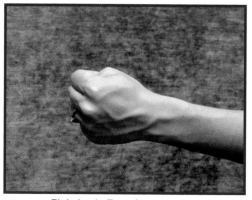

Finkelstein Test: Start Position

Hand &
Wrist

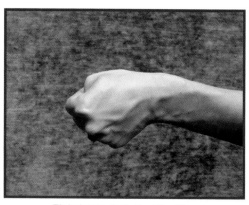

Finkelstein Test: End Position

Carpal Compression Test

Purpose:
To test for the presence of carpal tunnel syndrome.

Description:
The patient is seated with the forearm and hand to be tested resting on the table. The examiner applies compression over the carpal tunnel for 30 seconds.

Positive Test:
The test is considered positive if pain, parasthesias, or numbness is reproduced.

Diagnostic Accuracy:
Sensitivity = .42 - .75   - LR = .13 - .26[12-14 15]
Specificity = .84 - .95   + LR = 5.6 - 10.7[12-15]

Reliability:
Kappa = .77 (95% CI, .58, .96)[5]

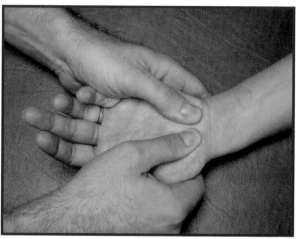

Carpal Compression Test

Clinical Prediction Rule for the Diagnosis of Carpal Tunnel Syndrome

Purpose:
To test for the presence of carpal tunnel syndrome.

Description:
A clinical prediction rule has been developed to identify the presence of carpal tunnel syndrome.[5] The rule consists of 5 predictor variables:

1. Age greater than 45
2. Patient reports shaking hands relieves symptoms
3. Wrist ratio index > .67
4. Reduced median sensory field of the first digit
5. Symptom Severity Scale score > 1.9

Patient reports shaking hands relieves symptoms:
This test is considered positive if the patient reports that symptoms improve with shaking or rapid alternating movements of the hand.
Reliability: ICC = .90[5]

Wrist ratio index:
A set of calipers is used to measure the anterior-posterior (AP) and medial-lateral (ML) wrist width. The wrist ratio index is calculated by dividing the AP by the ML wrist width. This criterion is satisfied if the index is > .67
Reliability: ICC = .77-.86[5]

Median Sensory Field 1:
Sensory testing is performed with the end of a straight paperclip. If sensation is reduced in the median sensory field of digit 1 as compared to the thenar eminence the test is considered positive.
Reliability: ICC = .48[5]

The Brigham and Women's Hospital Hand Severity Scale:
This criterion is satisfied if the Symptom Severity Score is ≥ 1.9.

Diagnostic Accuracy:
> 2 positive tests:	Sens= .98	Spec= .14	+LR= 1.1
> 3 positive tests:	Sens= .98	Spec= .54	+LR= 2.1
> 4 positive tests:	Sens= .77	Spec= .83	+LR= 4.6
If 5 positive tests:	Sens= .18	Spec= .99	+LR= 18.3

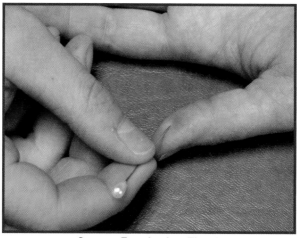

Sensory Examination: Thumb

Hand & Wrist

Reference List

(1) Cole IC. Fractures and ligament injuries of the wrist and hand. *The Wrist and Hand.*La, Crosse: Orthopaedic Section, American Physical Therapy Association; 1995.

(2) *Management of Common Musculoskeletal Disorders*. 3rd ed. Pennsylvania: Lippincott-Raven Publishers; 1996.

(3) Wadsworth C. Wrist and hand. *Current Concepts in Orthopaedic Physical Therapy.*La Crosse: Orthopaedic Section, American Physical Therapy Association; 2001.

(4) Wadsworth C. Cumulative trauma disorders of the wrist and hand. *The Wrist and Hand.*La Crosse: Orthopaedic Section, American Physical Therapy Association; 1995.

(5) Wainner RS, Fritz JM, Irrgang JJ, Delitto A, Allison S, Boninger ML. Development of a clinical prediction rule for the diagnosis of carpal tunnel syndrome. *Arch Phys Med Rehabil* 2005 April;86(4):609-18.

(6) Wolff TW, Hodges A. Common orthopaedic dysfunction of the wrist and hand. In: Placzek JD, Boyce DA, editors. Orthopaedic Physical Therapy Secrets. Philadelphia: Hanley and Belfus; 2001. p. 315-21.

(7) Horger M. The reliability of goniometric measurements of active and passive wrist motions. *Am J Occup Ther* 1990;44(4):342-8.

(8) Boone D, Azen S, Lin J, Baron C, et al. Reliability of goniometric measurements. *Phys Ther* 1978;58(11):1355-60.

(9) Brown A, Cramer LD, Eckhaus D, Schmidt J, Ware L, MacKenzie E. Validity and reliability of the dexter hand evaluation and therapy system in hand-injured patients. *J Hand Ther* 2000 January;13(1):37-45.

(10) Waeckerle JF. A prospective study identifying the sensitivity of radiographic findings and the efficacy of clinical findings in carpal navicular fractures. *Ann Emerg Med* 1987 July;16(7):733-7.

(11) LaStayo P, Howell J. Clinical provocative tests used in evaluating wrist pain: a descriptive study. *J Hand Ther* 1995 January;8(1):10-7.

(12) Szabo RM, Slater RR, Jr., Farver TB, Stanton DB, Sharman WK. The value of diagnostic testing in carpal tunnel syndrome. *J Hand Surg [Am]* 1999 July;24(4):704-14.

(13) Tetro AM, Evanoff BA, Hollstien SB, Gelberman RH. A new provocative test for carpal tunnel syndrome. Assessment of wrist flexion and nerve compression. *J Bone Joint Surg Br* 1998 May;80(3):493-8.

(14) Durkan JA. A new diagnostic test for carpal tunnel syndrome. *J Bone Joint Surg Am* 1991 April;73(4):535-8.

(15) Mondelli M, Passero S, Giannini F. Provocative tests in different stages of carpal tunnel syndrome. *Clin Neurol Neurosurg* 2001 October;103(3):178-83.

Hand & Wrist

TEMPOROMANDIBULAR EXAMINATION

In This Chapter:

1. **Historical Examination**
2. **Observation and Palpation**
3. **Active Range of Motion, Passive Range of Motion, and Overpressure**
   a. Mandibular Depression
   b. Lateral Deviation
   c. Protrusion and Retrusion
4. **Resisted Muscle Tests**
   a. Mandibular Depression
   b. Mandibular Elevation
   c. Lateral Deviation
5. **Assessment of Accessory Movements**
   a. Mandibular Distraction
   b. Anterior Glide of Mandible
   c. Lateral Glide of Mandible
6. **Special Tests**
   a. Auscultation during active movement

Region-Specific Historical Examination:

The patient should be asked specific questions related to the temporomandibular region and surrounding areas.

1. *Do you have limited opening of the mouth?*
   > If the patient answers "yes" this may indicate anterior disc displacement.[1-3]

2. *Do you have clicking during mouth opening and closing?*
   > If the patient answers "yes" this may indicate internal disc derangement.[1-3]

3. *Do you have creptius during mouth opening or closing?*
   > If the patient answers "yes" this may indicate an osteoarthritic condition of the temporomandibular joint.[4]

4. *Do yoursymptoms change (better or worse) with any movements of the neck?*
   > If the patient answers "yes" this indicates the cervical spine should be examined in detail.

5. *Does your jaw ever slip out or feel unstable?*
   > If the patient answers "yes" this may indicate possible mandibular subluxations.

TMD

Observation and Palpation:

This portion of the examination should be performed with the patient either standing or seated.

Observation

With the patient seated the examiner observes for any asymmetries in any of the soft tissues or bony landmarks.

Resting position of the mandible is observed.

The examiner should observe the patient from the anterior, posterior, and lateral views.

Palpation

The examiner palpates the temporomandibular joint, the masseter and temporalis muscles, and surround soft tissue structures. The examiner should also palpate for tenderness of the posterior occipital muscles.

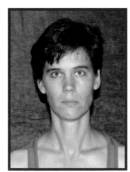
Anterior View

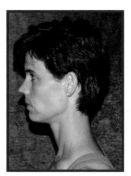
Lateral View

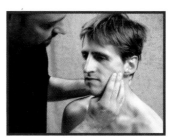
Masseter

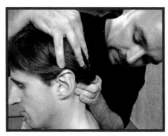
Posterior Occipital Muscles

TMD

Active Range of Motion, Passive Range of Motion, and Overpressure:

With the patient seated the examiner asks the patient to perform the following motions in order to assess the quality and quantity of motion and change in symptoms. Active range of motion can be quantified with a standard ruler. Following active range of motion testing the therapist moves the joint through maximal range of motion (as tolerated by the patient), applies overpressure, and assesses range of motion, pain reproduction, and end-feel.

Mandibular Depression

The patient is asked to open the mouth as far as possible. 40 mm is considered normal maximal mouth opening.[5] Overpressure can be applied at the end range of motion.

Reliability:

- Measurements of maximal mouth opening using a standard ruler have demonstrated an intra- rater reliability of .99 (ICC) and an inter-rater reliability of .94.[6]

Lateral Deviation

The patient is asked to laterally deviate the mandible as far as possible. Overpressure can be applied at the end range of motion.

Protrusion and Retrusion

The patient is asked to protrude and retrude the mandible. Overpressure can be applied at the end range of motion.

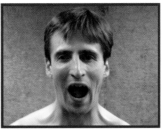

Maximal Mouth Opening

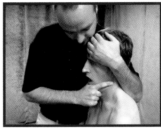

Maximal Mouth Opening with Overpressure

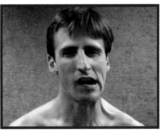

Lateral Deviation

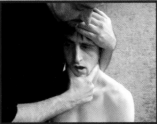

Lateral Deviation with Overpressure

TMD

Resisted Muscle Tests:

Resisted muscle tests are performed isometrically. They are included to assess strength of muscles and symptom response. The following list provides selected resisted tests that should be performed when examining the temporomandibular region.

Mandibular Depression

Seated, the patient is instructed to slightly depress the mandible. The examiner stabilizes the patient's head with one hand and then, in the direction of mouth closing, applies a superiorly directed force through the mandible.The patient is instructed to resist during this process.

Mandibular Elevation

Seated, the patient is instructed to slightly depress the mandible. The examiner stabilizes the patient's head with one hand and then applies an inferiorly directed force through the mandible, in the direction of mouth opening while the patient is instructed to resist.

Lateral Deviation

Seated, the patient is instructed to slightly depress the mandible. The examiner stabilizes the patient's head with one hand and then, in the direction of mouth opening applies a laterally directed force through the mandible. The patient is instructed to resist during this process.

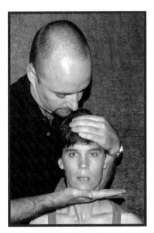

**Resisted Mandibular
Depression**

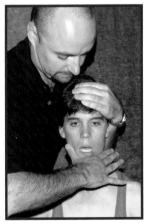

**Resisted Mandibular
Elevation**

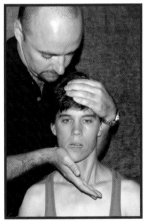

**Resisted Lateral
Deviation**

TMD

Assessments of Accessory Movements:

The examiner investigates accessory movement of the temporomandibular joint.

Mandibular Distraction

The examiner stands at the side of the patient and cradles the patient's head against the chest with one hand. The thumb and first finger of the opposite hand cradle the patient's mandible. The mandible is then distracted inferiorly while the examiner monitors the quality of movement and symptoms.

Anterior Glide of Mandible

The examiner stands at the side of the patient and cradles the patient's head against the chest with one hand. The thumb and first finger of the opposite hand cradle the patient's mandible. Slight distraction is applied to the joint then the examiner translates the mandible in an anterior direction while assessing the quality of movement and symptoms.

Lateral Glide of Mandible

The examiner stands at the side of the patient and cradles the patient's head against the chest with one hand. The thumb and first finger of the opposite hand cradle the patient's mandible. Slight distraction is applied to the joint then the examiner translates the mandible in a medial to lateral direction while assessing the quality of movement and symptoms.

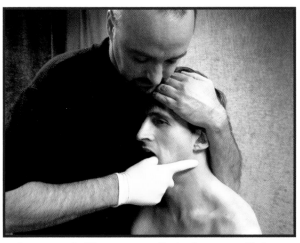

Assessment of Temporomandibular Accessory Motions

TMD

Special Tests:

Auscultation During Active Movement

Purpose:
To identify the presence of osteoarthritis of the temporomandibular joints.

Description:
The patient is seated and the examiner auscultates over both temporomandibular joints during mouth opening and closing.

Positive Test:
The test is considered positive if crepitus is heard by the examiner.

Diagnostic Accuracy:
Sensitivity = .45 - .67   - LR = .38 - .65
Specificity = .84 - .86   + LR = 2.8 - 4.8

Reliability:
Not reported

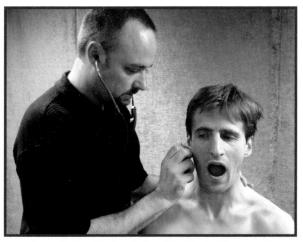

Auscultation During Active Mandibular Movement

Reference List

(1) Barclay P, Hollender L, Maravilla K, Truelove E. Comparison of clinical and magnetic resonance imaging diagnoses in patients with disk displacement in the temporomandibular joint. *Oral Surg Oral Med Oral Pathol* 1999;88:37-43.

(2) Cholitgul W, Nishiyama H, Sasai T, Uchiyama Y, Fuchihata H, Rohlin M. Clinical and magnetic resonance imaging findings in temporomandibular joint disc displacement. *Dentomaxillofacial Radiology* 1997;26:183-8.

(3) Orsini MG, Kuboki T, Terada S, Matsuka Y, Yatani H, Yamashita A. Clinical predictibility of temporomandibular joint disc displacement. *J Dent Res* 1999;78(2):650-60.

(4) Widmer CG. Evaluation of Temporomandibular Disorders. In: Kraus SL, editor. TMJ Disorders Management of the Craniomandibular Complex. New York: Churchill Livingstone; 1988. p. 79-112.

(5) Paesani D, Westesson PL, Hatala M, Tallents RH, Brooks S. Accuracy of clinical diagnosis for TMJ internal derangement and arthrosis. *Oral Surg Oral Med Oral Pathol* 1992;73:360-3.

(6) Walker N, Bohannon RW, Cameron D. Discriminant validity of temporomandibular joint range of motion measurements obtained with a ruler. *J Orthop Sports Phys Ther* 2000 August;30(8):484-92.

LUMBAR SPINE EXAMINATION

In This Chapter:

1. **Historical Examination & Visceral Referral Patterns**
2. **Observation, Functional Tests, & Palpation Active Range of Motion, Passive Range of Motion, and Overpressure**
    a. Flexion
    b. Extension
    c. Sidebending
    d. Combined Movements
3. **Resisted Muscle Tests**
    a. Flexion
    b. Extension
4. **Assessment of Accessory Movements**
    a. Posterior-Anterior Segmental Mobility
5. **Special Tests**
    a. Gillet Test
    b. Seated Flexion Test
    c. Slump Test
    d. Straight Leg Raise Test
    e. Posterior Shear Test (POSH)
    f. Gaenslen Test
    g. Flexion, Abduction, External Rotation Test (FABER or Patrick's Test)
    h. Spring Test
    i. Prone Instability Test (PIT)
    j. Test Item Cluster for Identification of Patients Likely to Benefit from Spinal Manipulation
    k. Test Item Cluster for Identification of Patients Likely to Benefit from Lumbar Stabilization Training

Lumbar
Spine

Region Specific Historical Examination:

In addition to the historical examination presented in Chapter three, the patient should be asked specific questions related to the lumbar spine and surrounding regions.

1. *Do your symptoms change (better or worse) with any movements of the neck or upper back?*
   If "yes" the cervical spine should be examined.

2. *The following questions have some utility in identifying patients with Lumbar Spinal Stenosis.*[1]

Question	+ LR (yes)	- LR (no)
Do you have *no* pain when sitting?	6.6	.58
Are your symptoms improved while seated?	3.1	.58
Age > 65	2.5	.33
Do you have severe lower extremity pain?	2.0	.52
Are you able to walk better when holding onto a shopping cart?	1.9	.55
Do you have pain below the knees?	1.5	.70
Do you have pain below the buttocks?	1.3	.35

3. *The following questions have some utility in identifying patients with Lumbar Zygapophyseal Pain Syndromes. If 5 of 7 are present it correctly identifies 92% of patients.*[3]

Question
1. Age > 65
2. Pain not worsened by coughing
3. Pain not worsened by hyperextension
4. Pain not worsened by forward flexion
5. Pain not worsened by extension-rotation
6. Pain not worsened when rising from a chair
7. *Pain relieved by recumbency (*must always be present)

4. *The following questions have limited utility in identifying patients with Lumbar Radiculopathy.*[4]

Question	+ LR (yes)	- LR (no)
Weakness	1.2	.73
Numbness	1.0	.94

5. *The following questions have limited utility in identifying patients with Ankylosing Spondylitis.*[5]

Question	+ LR (yes)	- LR (no)
Pain not relieved by lying down	1.6	.41
Morning stiffness > 1/2 hour	1.6	.68
Back pain at night	1.5	.55
Pain or stiffness relieved by exercise	1.3	.6
Age of onset < 40 years	1.1	0

Lumbar Spine

Observation

Watch the patient walk and observe any abnormal gait mechanics and/or reproduction of symptoms.

With the patient standing, the examiner observes for any asymmetries in any of the soft tissues or bony landmarks of the low back, hip, gluteal region, and lower extremities. The examiner should observe the patient from the anterior, posterior, and lateral views.

Functional Tests

The patient should demonstrate any functional movement or activity that reproduces symptoms. These functional movements often include one or more of the following activities:

- walking
- jogging
- hopping
- squatting
- donning/doffing socks & shoes
- transferring from sit to stand
- single leg stance
- crossing the legs while seated

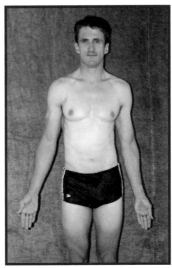

Anterior View

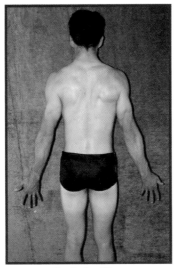

Posterior View

Palpation

The examiner palpates the lumbo-sacral, gluteal, and hip regions starting superficially and progressing to deeper structures. The examiner palpates for the presence of any temperature changes, moisture, soft tissue or lymph node swelling, and tissue texture abnormalities.

Symmetry of bony landmarks is observed including the iliac crests, ASIS, ischial tuberosities, and the region overlying the transverse processes.

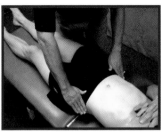

Iliac Crest

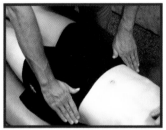

ASIS

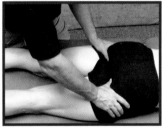

Ischial Tuberosities

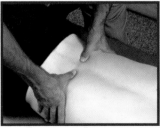

Transverse Processes

Lumbar
Spine

Active Range of Motion (AROM), Passive Range of Motion (PROM), and Overpressure:

With the patient standing, the examiner asks the patient to perform the following motions while assessing the quality and quantity of motion and change in symptoms, particularly if symptoms move distally from the spine ("peripheralization"). After performing active range of motion, the examiner passively moves the spine through maximal range of motion (as tolerated by the patient), applies overpressure, and assesses range of motion, pain reproduction, and end-feel. ROM can be quantified with a tape measure, standard goniometer or gravity/bubble inclinometer.

Flexion
Standing: The patient is asked to bend forward while keeping their knees straight. The quality of the motion is noted and the distance from the finger tips to the floor is measured. Overpressure can be applied at the end range of motion.

Extension
Standing: The patient is asked to bend backward while keeping the knees straight. The quality of the motion is noted. Overpressure can be applied at the end range of motion.

Sidebending
Standing: The patient is asked to bend sideways while keeping the knees straight. The quality of the motion is noted and the distance from the finger tips to the knee is measured. Overpressure can be applied at the end range of motion.

Combined Extension, Sidebending, Rotation (Quadrant)
Standing: The patient is asked to bend backward without bending the knees while reaching with the hands down the back of the legs. The quality of the motion is noted. Overpressure can be applied at the end range of motion.

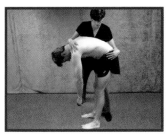

Flexion with Overpressure

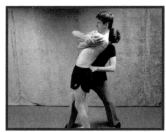

Extension with Overpressure

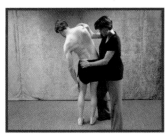

Sidebending with Overpressure

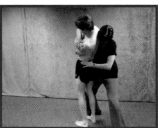

Combined with Overpressure

Lumbar
Spine

Resisted Muscle Tests:

Resisted muscle tests are performed isometrically and are performed to assess symptom response and strength. The following are selected resisted tests that can be performed when examining the lumbar region.

Flexion in Supine (Active Sit-Up Test)

The patient is supine and is asked to flex the knees to 90° and place the soles of the feet flat on the surface. The examiner holds both feet down with one hand. The patient is instructed to reach up with the fingertips of both hands to touch (not hold) both knees and hold the position for 5 seconds. If the patient cannot maintain this position for 5 seconds, the test is positive.

Extension in Prone (Extensor Endurance Test)

The patient is asked to lie prone while holding the sternum off the examination table for as long as possible. A small pillow is placed under the lower abdomen to decrease lumbar lordosis. The patient also needs to maintain maximum flexion of cervical spine and pelvic stabilization through gluteal contraction. The patient is asked to hold this position as long as possible not to exceed 5 minutes. The performance time is recorded in seconds.

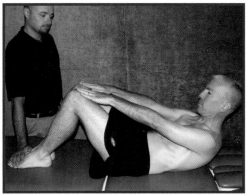

Active Sit-Up Test

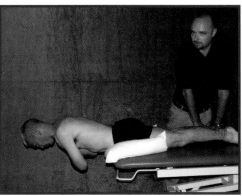

Extensor Endurance Test

Assessment of Accessory Movements

The examiner investigates accessory movement of the individual lumbar spine segments. With all tests, pain responses are recorded and mobility judgments are established as hypermobile, normal, or hypomobile.

Posteroanterior Mobility

Purpose:
To test for segmental movement and pain response.

Description:
The patient is prone. The examiner contacts the spinous process with the hypothenar eminence just distal to the pisiform. The examiner should be directly over the contact area and keep the elbows extended. The examiner uses the upper trunk to impart a posterior to anterior force in a progressive and oscillatory fashion over the spinous process. Repeat for remaining lumbar segments.

Positive Test:
The test result is considered to be positive if the patient reports reproduction of pain. The mobility of the segment is judged to be normal, hypermobile, or hypomobile.

Diagnostic Accuracy:
Lack of hypomobility during testing was related to radiographic lumbar instability.[6]
Sensitivity = .43   - LR = .60
Specificity = .95   + LR = 8.6

Reliability:
Kappa = 0.25 – 0.57 (pain) [7-9]
ICC = 0.25 – 0.77 (mobility) [7-9]

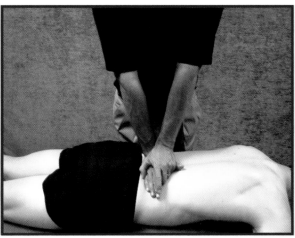

Posteroanterior Mobility

Special Tests:

Gillet Test

Purpose:
To test for the presence of motion restriction of the SI region.

Description:
The patient is standing. The examiner palpates the inferior aspect of the PSIS of tested side with one thumb and mid-point of sacrum (~S2) with the other thumb. The patient flexes the hip and the examiner judges if inferior and lateral movement of the tested PSIS occurs relative to the sacrum.

Positive Test:
The test is considered positive if there is no inferior movement of thumb on the PSIS.

Diagnostic Accuracy:
LR unknown

Reliability:
ICC = .59[10]

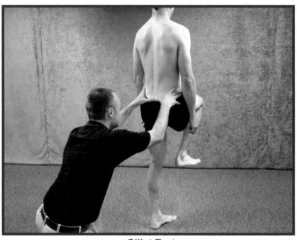

Gillet Test

Seated Flexion Test

Purpose:
To test for the presence of motion restriction of the SI region.

Description:
The patient is seated. The examiner's thumbs palpate the inferior aspect of each PSIS. The patient flexes forward while the examiner judges the movement of the PSIS. The examiner also observes the symmetry of movement in the lumbar spine.

Positive Test:
The test result is considered to be positive if more cephalad motion of one PSIS relative to the other PSIS occurs.

Diagnostic Accuracy:
Unknown

Reliability:
ICC = 0.25[10]

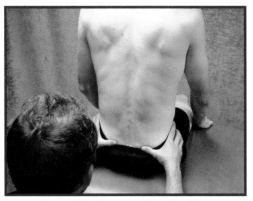

Seated Flexion Test: Start Position

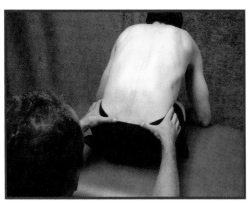

Seated Flexion Test: End Position

Lumbar
Spine

Slump Test

Purpose:
To test for the presence of sensitive neural tissue elements or altered neurodynamics as a possible source of symptoms.

Description:
The patient is seated in an upright posture with the hands clasped behind the back and knees together. The examiner introduces motions in this order:

>Spinal flexion
>Neck flexion
>Knee extension
>Release neck flexion

Positive Test:
The test result is considered to be positive if symptoms decrease with release of neck flexion.

Diagnostic Accuracy:
Not Reported

Reliability:
Not Reported

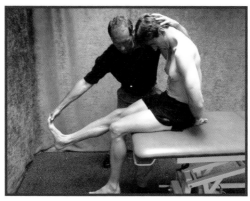

Slump Test: Start Position

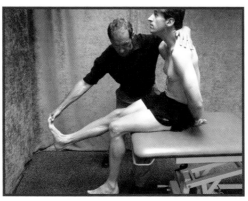

Slump Test: End Position

Lumbar
Spine

Straight Leg Raise

Purpose:
To test for the presence of disk herniation.

Description:
The patient is supine, the knee is fully extended, and ankle is in neutral dorsiflexion. The examiner passively flexes the hip while maintaining the knee in extension. The amount of hip flexion is recorded at the point of pain or in paresthesia the back or lower limb.

Positive Test:
The test result is considered to be positive if the patient reports reproduction of back or leg pain at 40 degrees or less.

Diagnostic Accuracy:
Sensitivity = .91   - LR = .35
Specificity = .26   + LR = 1.2

Crossed Straight Leg Raise:
The test entails performing the straight leg raise test on the uninvolved extremity. It is considered positive if it reproduces symptoms in the involved extremity.

Diagnostic Accuracy:
Sensitivity = .29   - LR = .80[11]
Specificity = .88   + LR = 2.4[11]

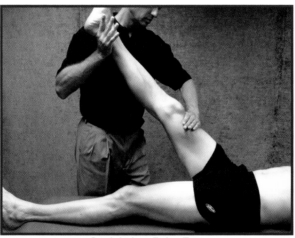

Straight Leg Raise Test

Posterior Shear (POSH) Test

Purpose:
To test for pain of sacroiliac origin.

Description:
The patient is supine, the knee and hip are flexed to 90 degrees. The examiner places a hand underneath the sacrum. The examiner delivers a posterior directed force through the femur at varying angles of abduction/adduction.

Positive Test:
The test result is considered to be positive if buttock pain is reproduced.

Diagnostic Accuracy:
Reference standard anesthetic block of the sacroiliac joint

Sensitivity = .80   - LR = .2[12]

Specificity = 1.0   + LR = NA[12]

Reliability:
Inter-examiner Kappa = 0.64 - 0.88[10,14]

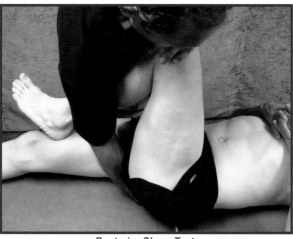

Posterior Shear Test

Gaenslen Test

Purpose:
To test for pain of sacroiliac origin.

Description:
The patient is supine with both legs extended. The leg being tested is passively brought into full knee flexion, while the opposite hip remains in extension. Overpressure is then applied to the flexed extremity.

Positive Test:
The test result is considered to be positive if the patient reports reproduction of pain in the lower back.

Diagnostic Accuracy:
Reference standard anesthetic block of the sacroiliac joint
Sensitivity = .71   - LR = 1.12[12]
Specificity = .26   + LR = 1.0[12]

Reliability:
Inter-examiner Kappa = 0.54 - 0.76[10,14]

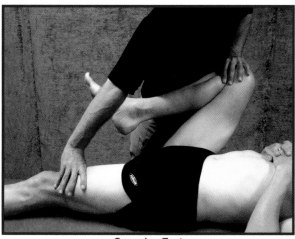

Gaenslen Test

Flexion, Abduction, External Rotation Test
(FABER or Patrick's Test)

Purpose:
To test for the presence of sacroiliac region pain; also, to test for the presence of hip pathology

Description:
The patient is supine. The tested LE is placed in a "figure 4" position (hip flexed and abducted, ipsilateral foot resting on the contralateral thigh just above the knee). While stabilizing the opposite side of the pelvis, an external rotation / posteriorly directed force is then applied to the ipsilateral knee.

Positive Test:
The test result is considered to be positive if the patient reports reproduction of buttock or groin pain.

Diagnostic Accuracy:
Reference standard anesthetic block of the sacroiliac joint
Sensitivity = .71   - LR = .23[12]
Specificity = 1.0   + LR = NA[12]

Reliability:
Inter-examiner Kappa = 0.60 - 0.62[10,14]

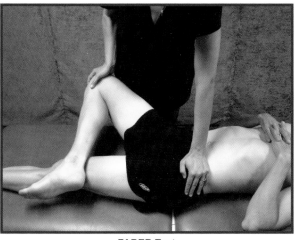

FABER Test

Lumbar
Spine

Resisted Abduction Test

Purpose:
To test for pain of sacroiliac origin.

Description:
The patient is supine with the leg fully extended and abducted to 30 degrees. The examiner then resists abduction.

Positive Test:
The test result is considered to be positive if the patient reports reproduction of low back pain.

Diagnostic Accuracy:
Reference standard anesthetic block of the sacroiliac joint
Sensitivity = .87   - LR = .13[12]
Specificity = 1.0   + LR = NA[12]

Reliability:
Not Reported

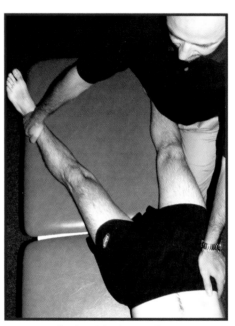

Resisted Abduction Test

Prone Instability Test (PIT)

Purpose:
To test for the likelihood of a patient responding to a stabilization exercise program.

Description:
The patient lies prone with the body on the examining table and legs over the edge and feet resting on the floor. While the patient rests in this position, the examiner applies posterior to anterior pressure to the lumbar spine. Any provocation of pain is reported. Then the patient lifts the legs off the floor (the patient may hold table to maintain position) and posterior compression is applied again to the lumbar spine.

Positive Test:
The test result is considered to be positive if pain is present in the resting position but subsides in the second position.

Diagnostic Accuracy:
Reference standard success with stabilization exercise program.

Sensitivity = .72   - LR = .48[7]
Specificity = .58   + LR = 1.7[7]

Reliability:
Not Reported

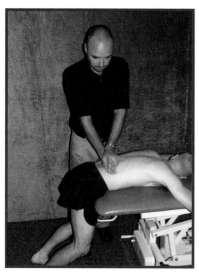

Prone Instability Test: Start

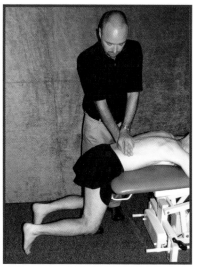

Prone Instability Test: End

Lumbar
Spine

Test Item Cluster for Patients Likely to Benefit from Spinal Manipulation

Purpose:
To determine the likelihood of patients responding with a 50% or greater reduction in disability following a program of spinal manipulation and exercise.

Description:
The following test item clusters can be performed entirely in the history and physical exam without any additional lab or imaging tests.

Test Items:

Criterion Definition of Positive:
- Duration of current episode of low back pain 16 days or less
- Not having symptoms distal to the knee
- FABQ work subscale score 18 points or less
- Segmental mobility testing noting at least 1 hypomobile segment in the lumbar spine
- Hip internal rotation range of motion with 1 or both hips having at least 35 degrees of internal rotation

Diagnostic Accuracy:
Reference standard for success with spinal manipulation.
When at least 4 of of the 5 criteria were met: + LR = 13.2[15]
When only 1 or 2 of the criteria were met: - LR = .10[15]

Test Item Cluster for Patients Likely to Benefit from Lumbar Stabilization Exercise Training

Purpose:
To determine the likelihood of patients responding with a 50% or greater reduction in disability following a program of lumbar spine stabilization exercises.

Description :
The following test item clusters can be performed entirely in the history and physical exam without any additional lab or imaging tests.

Test Items:

Criterion Definition of Positive:
- Age less than 40 years
- Average SLR >91°
- Positive prone instability test
- Aberrant movement present (Examined during lumbar ROM testing). Described as an instability catch, painful arc of motion, "thigh climbing" (Gower's sign), or a reversal of lumbopelvic rhythm.

Diagnostic Accuracy:
Reference standard for success with a program of lumbar spine stabilization exercises.

When at least 3 of the 4 criteria were met: + LR = 4.0[7]

When only 1 of 4 of the criteria was met: - LR = .20[7]

When only 2 of 4 of the criteria were met: - LR = .30[7]

Reference List

(1)   Katz JN Dalgas M, Stucki G et al. Degenerative lumbar spinal stenosis. Diagnostic value of the history and physical examination. *Arthiris Rheum* 1995; 38:1236-41.

(2)   Fritz JM, Whitman JM, Childs JD. Lumbar spine segmental mobility assessment: an examination of validity for determining intervention strategies in patients with low back pain. *Arch Phys Med Rehabil* 2005;86:1745-1752.

(3)   Revel M, Poiraudeau S, Auleley G, et al. Capacity of the clinical picture to characterize low back pain relieved by facet joint anesthesia: Proposed criteria to identify patients with painful facet joints. *Spine* 1998;23:1972-1976.

(4)   Lauder T, Dillingham T, Andary M, et al. Effect of history and exam in predicting electrodiagnostic outcome among patients with suspected lumbosacral radiculopathy. *Am J Phys Med* 2000;79:60-68.

(5)   Gran J. An epidemiological survey of the signs and symptoms of ankylosing spondylitis. *Clin Rheumatol* 1985;4:161-169.

(6)   Fritz JM, Piva SR, Childs JD. Accuracy of the clinical examination to predict radiographic instability of the lumbar spine. *Eur Spine J* 2005;14:743-750.

(7)   Hicks G, Fritz J, Delitto A, McGill S. Preliminary development of a clinical prediction rule for determining which patients with low back pain will respond to a stabilization exercise program. *Arch Phys Med Rehabil* 2005;86:1753-1762.

(8)   Binkley J, Stratford P, Gill C. Interrater reliability of lumbar accessory motion mobility testing. *Phys Ther* 1995;75:786-795.

(9)   Maher C, Latimer J, Adams R. An investigation of the reliability and validity of posteroanterior spinal stiffness judgments made using a reference-based protocol. *Phys Ther* 1998;78:829-837.

(10) Flynn T, Fritz J, Whitman J, et al. A clinical prediction rule for classifying patients with low back pain who demonstrate short-term improvement with spinal manipulation. *Spine* 2002;27:2835-2843.

(11) Deville W, van der Windt D, Dzaferagic A, et al. The test of Lasègue. Systematic review of the accuracy in diagnosing herniated discs. *Spine* 2000;25:1140-1147.

(12) Broadhurst N, Bond M. Pain provocation tests for the assessment of sacroiliac joint dysfunction. *J Spinal Disorders* 1998;11:341-345.

(13) Dreyfuss P, Michaelsen M, Pauza K, et al. The value of medical history and physical examination in diagnosing sacroiliac joint pain. *Spine* 1996;21:2594-2602.

(14) Laslett M, Williams M. The reliability of selected pain provocation tests for sacroiliac joint pathology. *Spine* 1994;19:1243-1249.

(15) Childs JD, Fritz JM, Flynn TW, et al. A clinical prediction rule to identify patients with low back pain most likely to benefit from spinal manipulation: a validation study. *Ann Intern Med* 2004;141:920-928.

Lumbar
Spine

HIP EXAMINATION

In This Chapter:

1. **Historical Examination & Visceral Referral Patterns**
2. **Observation, Functional Tests, & Palpation**
3. **Active Range of Motion, Passive Range of Motion, & Overpressures**
   a. Flexion
   b. Internal Rotation and External Rotation
   c. Abduction and Adduction
   d. Extension
4. **Resisted Muscle Tests**
   a. Flexion
   b. Abduction
   c. Internal Rotation and External Rotation
   d. Extension
5. **Muscle Length/Flexibility**
   a. Iliopsoas
   b. Rectus Femoris
   c. Hamstrings
   d. Tensor Fascia Latae / IT Band
   e. Piriformis > 90° Flexion
   f. Piriformis < 90° Flexion
6. **Assessments of Accessory Movements**
   a. Inferior Glide
   b. Posterior Glide
   c. Lateral Glide
   d. Long-Axis Distraction
   e. Anterior Glide
7. **Special Tests**
   a. Flexion, Abduction, External Rotation Test (or FABER or Patrick's Test)
   b. Test Item Cluster for Identification of Hip Osteoarthritis
   c. Flexion, Adduction, Internal Rotation, and Compression Test (or Quadrant Test)
   d. Limited Hip Abduction Test
   e. Flexion, Adduction, Internal Rotation (FAIR) Test

Hip

Region Specific Historical Examination:

In addition to the historical examination presented in Chapter 3, the patient should be asked specific questions related to the hip and surrounding regions.

1. *Do your symptoms change (better or worse) with any movements of the low back? Do you have any pain in your low back, even if you feel it is unrelated to your hip pain?*

   If the patient answers "yes" for either question, the lumbar spine and pelvis should be examined in addition to the hip.

2. *Does your hip pain extend down into your thigh or leg? Do you ever experience numbness or tingling into the hip, thigh, leg, ankle, or foot?*

   If the patient answers "yes" for either question, both a LE neurological screening examination and a lumbar spine examination should be performed to identify any existing radiculopathy or radiculitis.

   If symptoms refer into the posterior thigh and perhaps the calf without numbness/tingling without numbness or tingling, the following diagnoses should be considered: Ischial bursitis[1], Hamstring strain[1], Piriformis syndrome.[2]

3. *Have you recently increased your physical activity, especially running (distance, terrain, speed) or other weight bearing activities?*

   If the patient answers "yes" the clinician should be suspicious of a femoral neck, femoral shaft, or pelvic stress reaction or stress fracture.[3] Muscle sprain/strain should also be considered.[1]

4. *Do you have pain or stiffness in the hip or groin region? Do you have a family history of osteoarthritis? Morning stiffness < 60 minutes? Pain with prolonged walking?*

   If the patient answers "yes" the clinician should be suspicious of hip osteoarthritis.[4]

5. *Do you experience clicking, catching, or giving way of the hip? Do your symptoms worsen with full flexion or extension?*

   If the patient answers "yes" a labral lesion or tear[5,6] should be considered.

Other conditions to consider based on the historical exam:

If the patient is young (age 4-6 yrs) with hip, groin, thigh, or knee pain, Legg-Calvé-Perthes disease should be considered.[7;8] This condition occurs more often in females than males, and these children tend to be smaller and fairly physically active.

If the patient is a young adolescent (age 11-14 years) with insidious onset of hip, groin, thigh, or knee pain, slipped capital femoral epiphysis should be considered.[7,9] This condition occurs more often in males than females, and these children tend to be overweight.

A history of aching and/or deep throb in the groin or hip region combined with a history of prolonged steroid use, excessive alcohol use, blood disorders, or chemotherapy or radiation should lead the clinician to consider avascular necrosis or osteonecrosis as a possible diagnosis.[5]

Pain extending along the lateral thigh, and exacerbated with ascending/descending stairs or transferring from sit to stand may be indicative of greater trochanteric bursitis[10] or a muscle strain[1].

Hip

Observation

Watch the patient walk and observe any abnormal gait mechanics and/or reproduction of symptoms.

With the patient standing, the examiner observes for any asymmetries in any of the soft tissues or bony landmarks of the hip, gluteal region, low back, and lower extremities. The examiner should observe the patient from the anterior, posterior, and lateral views.

Functional Tests

The patient should demonstrate any functional movement or activity that reproduces symptoms. These functional movements often include one or more of the following activities: walking, jogging, hopping, squatting, donning/doffing socks & shoes, transferring from sit to stand, single leg stance, and crossing the legs while seated.

These tests allow for a quick functional screen of the patient's entire lower quarter. Appropriate selection of the tests should be based on the patient's age, activity level, and severity of pain. The clinician should assess the quality and quantity of motion and any change in symptoms with test performance.

Palpation

The examiner palpates the hip, gluteal, and lumbo-sacral regions starting superficially and progressing to deeper structures. The examiner palpates for the presence of any temperature changes, moisture, soft tissue or lymph node swelling, and tissue texture abnormalities.

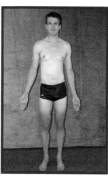
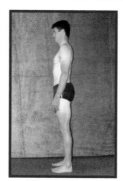
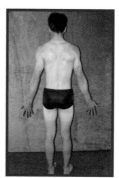

Anterier View   **Lateral View**   **Posterior View**

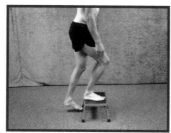
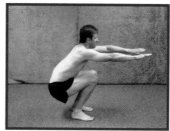

Functional Test:
Step Up

Functional Test:
Squat

Hip

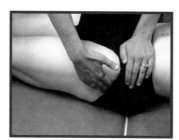
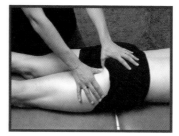

Palpation

Active Range of Motion (AROM), Passive Range of Motion (PROM), & Overpressure:

With the patient supine, the examiner asks the patient to perform the following motions while assessing the quality and quantity of motion and change in symptoms. After performing active range of motion, the examiner passively moves the joint through maximal range of motion (as tolerated by the patient), applies overpressure, and assesses range of motion, pain reproduction, and end-feel. ROM can be quantified with a standard goniometer or gravity/bubble inclinometer.

Flexion

The patient is asked to bring the knee up toward the chest. While maintaining the hip in neutral rotation, and without allowing the hip to abduct/adduct, the clinician moves the hip through full passive flexion range of motion. Overpressure can be applied at the end range of motion.

Internal Rotation (IR) and External Rotation (ER)

The patient's hip is placed in 90 degrees flexion and 0 degrees of abduction/adduction. While maintaining these positions, the clinician performs full passive internal and external rotation of the hip. Overpressure can be applied at the end range of motion.

Alternate technique with the patient in sitting: Stabilize the knee to prevent hip abduction/adduction and ask the patient to bring the foot up and out (external rotation) and up and in (internal rotation). While stabilizing the knee with one hand, the clinician can use the other hand to perform PROM and to apply overpressure.

Abduction and Adduction

The patient is asked to slide the hip away from midline as far as possible. While stabilizing the pelvis, the clinician passively abducts the hip through full range of motion. Next, with the opposite hip abducted approximately 30 degrees and the pelvis stabilized by the clinician, the patient is asked to bring the hip towards the opposite hip (adduction). The clinician can then passively adduct the hip through full range of motion. Overpressure can be applied at the end range of motion.

Extension

Prone: While keeping the knee extended and back straight, the patient should raise the knee up toward the ceiling as far as possible. The examiner then grasps the distal thigh (while supporting the leg), applies a posterior-to-anterior directed force over the ischial tuberosity to stabilize the pelvis, and extends the hip through full passive range of motion. Overpressure can be applied at the end range of motion.

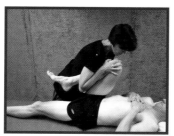

Flexion with Overpressure

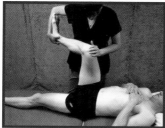

Internal Rotation with Overpressure

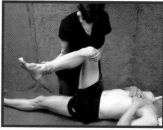

External Rotation with Overpressure

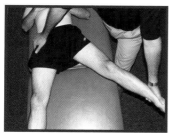

Abduction with Overpressure

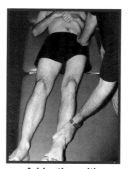

Adduction with Overpressure

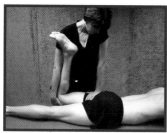

Extension with Overpressure

Hip

Resisted Muscle Tests:

Resisted tests are performed isometrically and are performed to assess symptom response and strength. The following list provides selected resisted tests that should be performed when examining the hip region.

Flexion in Sitting or Supine

Sitting: The examiner asks the patient to sit upright and to lift the knee 8 – 10 cm from the table. While stabilizing the patient's trunk/pelvis, the patient is then asked to resist an inferiorly directed force produced by the examiner through the patient's distal thigh.

Supine: The examiner asks the patient to keep the knee straight and to lift the leg approximately 30°. The patient is then asked to resist an inferiorly directed force produced by the examiner through the leg or distal thigh.

Abduction in Side-Lying or Supine

Side-lying: While stabilizing the pelvis, the examiner asks the patient to bring the leg up toward the ceiling. The patient is then asked to resist an inferiorly force produced by the examiner through the patient's distal lateral thigh. Note: Ensure that the patient does not flex the hip while performing the test.

Supine: While stabilizing the opposite LE, the patient is asked to slide the tested LE outward and then resist a medially directed force produced by the examiner through the lower leg.

Hip Internal Rotation and External Rotation in Sitting

Internal Rotation: With the hip positioned in internal rotation and the examiner stabilizing the medial knee, the patient is asked to resist a medially directed force applied to the lateral lower leg.

External Rotation: With the hip positioned in external rotation and the examiner stabilizing the lateral knee, the patient is asked to resist a laterally directed force applied to the medial lower leg.

Hip Extension in Prone

The examiner asks the patient to keep the knee straight and to lift the leg approximately 10°. The patient is then asked to resist an inferiorly directed force produced by the examiner through the leg or distal thigh. Note: To preferentially assess the gluteal musculature (vs hamstrings), position the knee in flexion while testing hip extension.

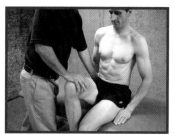

Resisted Flexion

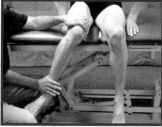

Resisted Internal Rotation

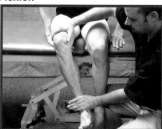

Resisted External Rotation

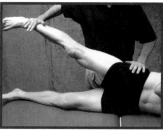

Resisted Abduction

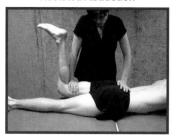

Resisted Extension

Hip

Muscle Length/Flexibility:

These tests are performed to assess the length and/or flexibility of the hip and gluteal region musculature. The following list provides selected resisted tests that should be performed when examining this region. Muscle length can often be quantified with a standard goniometer or gravity/bubble inclinometer.

Iliopsoas

Supine: Flex the hips and knees until the lumbar spine is flat against the table. While maintaining the non-tested LE in this position, slowly lower the tested LE toward the floor by extending the hip. The final resting position of the hip can be measured to quantitatively assess iliopsoas muscle length. For normal length, the thigh should lie parallel to the treatment table, or fall below the level of the treatment table.

Prone: Stabilize the patient's ischeal tuberosity with one hand (apply posterior-to-anterior directed force) and passively extend the patient's hip with the other. You should be able to extend the hip at least 10°.

Rectus Femoris

Prone: Stabilize the patient's ischeal tuberosity with one hand (apply posterior-to-anterior directed force) and passively flex the patient's knee. Keep the hip in midline while performing this test and don't allow either hip to flex.

Hamstrings

Supine: While keeping the non-tested LE stabilized against the table, flex the hip of the tested LE to 90°. Have the patient help you maintain 90° hip flexion while passively extending passively extend the knee. While no normative data are available, many clinicians feel the hamstrings are tight if the patient lacks 10°-20° to reach full extension with this test.

Tensor Fascia Latae and Iliotibial Band (Ober's Test)

Sidelying: Stabilize the patient's pelvis. Flex the underlying LE slightly to help stabilize the patient in sidelying. Flex the knee and hip of the tested LE (upper LE), passively abduct the hip, then extend the hip until the thigh is in line Keep the knee flexed to 90° while lowering the thigh. If the hip remains abducted (does not adduct beyond horizontal), then the patient has tightness of the TFL and ITB.

Piriformis at > 90 degrees flexion

Supine: Externally rotate and flex the hip. Add to the stretch by adducting the hip toward the opposite shoulder.

Piriformis at < 90 degrees flexion

Supine: Place the foot of the tested LE lateral to the knee or distal thigh of the non-tested LE. Stabilize the pelvis on the tested side, and bring the knee slowly towards and across midline.

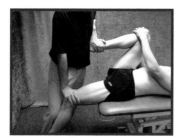

Iliopsoas

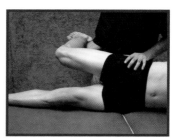

Rectus Femoris

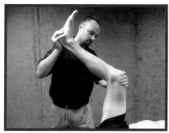

Hamstrings

Tensor Fascia Latae
& Iliotibial Band

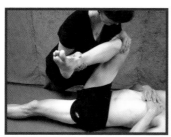

Piriformis above 90° Flexion

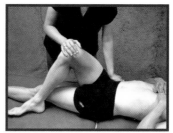

Piriformis below 90° Flexion

Hip

Assessment of Accessory Movements

The examiner investigates accessory movement of the hip joint in supine and prone. With all tests pain responses are recorded, and mobility judgments are established as hypermobile, normal, or hypomobile.

Inferior Glide of the Femur

Supine: Flex the hip passively to 90°. Grasp the proximal femur as shown, apply an inferiorly directed force to the most proximal aspect of the femur.

Posterior Glide of the Femur

Supine: Passively flex the hip to 90°. With the hip internally rotated and adducted, the examiner applies a posteriorly directed force through the femur.

Lateral Glide of the Femur

Supine: Passively flex the hip to 90°, grasp the proximal femur as shown, and apply a laterally directed force to the most proximal aspect of the femur.

Long-Axis Distraction of the Hip Joint

Supine: Grasp the patient's ankle, passively flex the hip 20°-30°, abduct approximately 30°, and apply a longitudinal distraction force to the hip.

Anterior Glide of the Femur

Prone: Fully extend the patient's hip and apply a posterior-to-anterior directed force over the proximal femur (either just inferior to the ischial tuberosity or over the posterior aspect of the greater trochanter). It may be easier to handle the leg if the knee is flexed while performing the test.

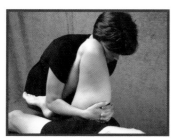

Inferior Glide

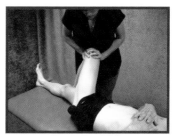

Posterior Glide

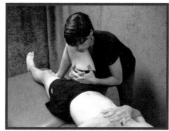

Lateral Glide

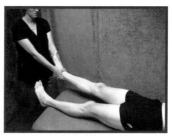

Long Axis Distraction

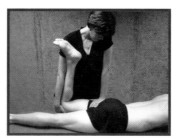

Anterior Glide

Hip

Special Tests:

Flexion, Abduction, External Rotation Test

(FABER or Patrick's Test)

Purpose:
To test for the presence of hip pathology.

Description:
The patient is supine. The tested LE is placed in a "figure 4" position (hip flexed and abducted, ipsilateral foot resting on the contralateral thigh just above the knee). While stabilizing the opposite side of the pelvis, an external rotation / posteriorly directed force is then applied to the ipsilateral knee.

Positive Test:
The test result is considered to be positive if the patient reports reproduction of hip pain in this position,[11] or if there is a restriction of ROM.[12]

Diagnostic Accuracy:
Sn (for identification of hip pathology identified with arthroscopy) = 0.89
LRs and Sp = unable to calculate[11]

Correlation of positive test with OA on radiographs: r = 0.54[12]

Reliability:
ICC = 0.66 - 0.96[12, 13]

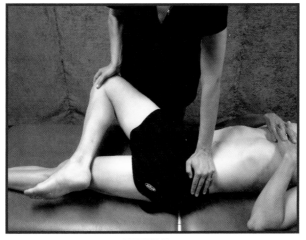

FABER Test

Hip

Test Item Cluster for the Identification of Hip Osteoarthritis

Purpose:
To test the presence of hip osteoarthritis.

Description:
The following test item clusters can be performed entirely in the history and physical examination without any additional lab or imaging tests.

Test Cluster 1:
1. Hip pain
2. Hip internal rotation range of motion <15°
3. Hip flexion range of motion <115° deg.

If hip internal rotation range of motion is > 15°, then use the following test cluster:

Test Cluster 2:
1. Painful hip with hip internal rotation
2. >50 years of age
3. Morning hip stiffness < 60 minutes

Diagnostic Accuracy:
Test Clusters 1 & 2
If all three components of a test cluster are present: + LR = 3.4[4]
If all 3 are not met: - LR = 0.19[4]

Reliability:
Not reported

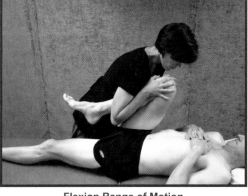

Flexion Range of Motion

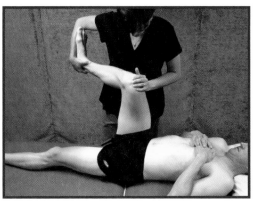

Internal Rotation Range of Motion

Hip

Flexion, Adduction, Internal Rotation, and Compression Test (Hip Quadrant)

Purpose
To test for the presence of hip pathology.

Description
With the patient in supine, the tested LE is passively flexed and adducted until resistance to movement is detected. The examiner then maintains flexion into resistance and moves the hip into abduction, bringing the hip through a full arc of motion. If the patient reports no pain, the examiner then applies long-axis compression to the hip through the femur.

Positive Test:
The test result is considered to be positive if the patient reports reproduction of hip pain in this position, or if there is a restriction of ROM.

Diagnostic Accuracy
Diagnostic characteristics for detection of acetabular labral lesions[6]
Sensitivity = .75   - LR = .58
Specificity = .43   + LR = 1.32

Reliability
ICC = .87[13]

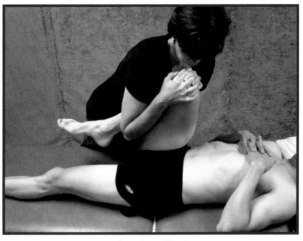

Quadrant Test

Flexion, Adduction, Internal Rotation (FAIR) Test [2,14]

Purpose
To detect compression or irritation of the sciatic nerve by the piriformis.

Description
With the patient in side-lying (non-tested LE is closest to the table), the patient's involved LE is passively brought into a position of flexion, adduction, and internal rotation.

Positive Test:
Pain detected at the region of the piriformis.

Diagnostic Accuracy
Sensitivity = .88 $- LR = .14^{2,14}$
Specificity = .83 $+ LR = 5.2^{2,14}$

Reliability
Not Reported

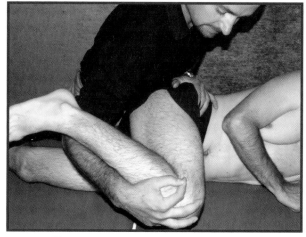

Flexion, Adduction, Internal Rotation Test

Hip

Reference List

(1)   Pecina MM, Bojanic I. *Overuse* Injuries of the Musculoskeletal System. Boca Raton: CRC Press; 1993.

(2)   Fishman L, Dombi G, Michaelson C, Ringel S, Rozbruch J, Rosner B et al. Piriformis syndrome: Diagnosis, treatment and outcome- a 10-year study. *Arch Phys Med Rehabil* 2002; 83:295-301.

(3)   O'Kane JW.   Anterior hip pain. *Am Fam Physician* 1999; 60(6):1687-1696.

(4)   Altman R, Alarcon G, Appelrouth D, Bloch D, Borenstein D, Brandt K et al. The American College of Rheumatology criteria for the classification and reporting of osteoarthritis of the hip. *Arth Rheum* 1991; 34(5):505-514.

(5)   Hartley A. Practical Joint Assessment. *St Louis: Mosby*, 1995.

(6)   Narvani A, Tsirdis E, Kendall S, Chaudhuri R, Thomas P. A preliminary report on prevalence of acetabular labral tears in sports patients with groin pain. *Knee Surg Sports Traumatol Arthrosc* 2003; 11:403-408.

(7)   Weinstein SL. Natural history and treatment outcomes of childhood hip disorders. *Clin Ortho Rel Rsch* 1997; 344:227-242.

(8)   Scherl SA. Common lower extremity problems in children. *Pediatrics in Review* 2004; 25(2):52-62.

(9)   Reynolds RA. Diagnosis and treatment of slipped capital femoral epiphysis. *Current Opinion in Pediatrics* 1999; 11(1):80-83.

(10)   Hertling D, Kessler RM. The hip. In: Hertling D, Kessler RM, editors. Management of Common Musculoskeletal Disorders: Physical Therapy Principles and Methods. *3rd ed. Philadelphia: Lippincott*, 1996. 285-314.

(11)   Mitchell B, McCroy P, Brukner P, O'Donnell J, Colson E, Howells R. Hip joint pathology: Clinical presentation and correlation between magnetic resonance arthrography, ultrasound, and arthroscopic findings in 25 consecutive cases. *Clin J Sports Med* 2003; 13:152-156.

(12)   Theiler R, Stucki G, Schotz R, Hofer H, Seifert B, Tyndall A et al. Parametric and non-parametric measures in the assessment of knee and hip osteoarthritis: interobserver reliability and correlation with radiology. *Osteoarthritis Cartilage* 1996;35-42.

(13) Cliborne A, Wainner R, Rhon D, Judd C, Fee T, Matekel R et al. Clinical hip tests and a functional squat test in patients with knee osteoarthritis: Reliability, prevalence of positive test findings, and short-term response to hip mobilization. *J Orthop Sports Phys Ther* 2004; 34:676-685.

(14) Jari S, Paton R, Srinivasan M. Unilateral limitation of abduction of the hip: A valuable clinical sign for DDH? *J Bone Joint Surg* 2002; 84-B:104-107.

(15) Fishman L, Zybert P. Electrophysiologic evidence of piriformis syndrome. *Arch Phys Med Rehabil* 1992; 73:359-364.

Hip

KNEE EXAMINATION

In This Chapter:

Knee

Region Specific Historical Examination:

In addition to the historical examination presented in Chapter three, the patient should be asked specific questions related to the knee and surrounding regions.

1. ***Do your symptoms change (better or worse) with any movements of the low back? Do you have any pain in your low back, even if you feel it is unrelated to your knee pain?***

    If "yes" for either question, the lumbo-pelvic region and hip should be examined in addition to the knee.

2. ***Does your knee pain extend up into your thigh or back or down into the leg, ankle, or foot? Do you ever experience numbness or tingling into the hip, thigh, leg, ankle, or foot?***

    If "yes" for either question, both a LE neurological screening examination and a lumbar spine examination should be performed to identify any existing radiculopathy or radiculitis.

    If symptoms are reported in the posterior thigh and perhaps the calf, but no numbness/tingling, the following diagnoses should be considered: Ischial bursitis[1] , Hamstring strain1,Piriformis syndrome[2].

3. ***Have you recently increased your physical activity, especially running (distance, terrain, speed) or other weight bearing activities?***

    If "yes", the clinician should be suspicious of a femoral, tibial, or fibular stress reaction or stress fracture. Muscle sprain/strain should also be considered.

4. ***Do you have knee pain or stiffness that eases after a few hours in the morning?***

    If "yes", the clinician should be suspicious of knee osteoarthritis.[3,4]

5. ***Is your knee pain a result of trauma, such as injury with jumping/landing, changing directions with your foot planted, or twisting?***

    If "yes", the following diagnoses should be considered: ligamentous injury, patellar subluxation, quadriceps rupture, meniscal lesion.[5-8]

    If the injury described resulted in a posteriorly directed blow to the tibia with the knee flexed, the clinician should consider possible posterior cruciate ligament injury.[5]

    If the injury described resulted in a valgus or varus stress to the knee, collateral ligament injury (fibular or tibial) should be considered.[5]

Other conditions to consider based on the historical exam:

If the patient complains of anterior knee pain that worsens with jumping, full knee flexion, or other activities that stress the extensor mechanism of the knee, patellar tendonitis[7,9] and patellofemoral pain syndrome[10,11] (also called retropatellar pain syndrome and anterior knee pain) should be considered. If the patient is young, and if the pain is localized to the insertion of the patellar tendon at the tibial tuberosity, Osgood-Schlater's Disease should also be considered.[12]

Patient reports of anterior knee pain that worsens with prolonged knee flexion ("positive movie sign"), squatting, and going up/down stairs should prompt the clinician to consider patellofemoral pain syndrome as a diagnosis.[10,11]

A patient complaint of knee swelling and knee locking and/or clicking should prompt the clinician to consider a meniscal lesion[8] or a possible loose body within the knee.

Lumbo-pelvic and hip conditions can be the source of referred pain to the knee. Incorporation of pertinent historical exam questions with physical exam tests from the Lumbar Spine and Hip Chapters will enhance the clinician's knee examination.

Knee

Observation, Functional Quick Tests, and Palpation:

Observation

Watch the patient walk and observe abnormal gait mechanics and/or reproduction of symptoms.

With the patient standing, the examiner observes for any asymmetries in any of the soft tissues or bony landmarks of the lumbo-pelvic region and lower extremities. For patients with knee pain, the clinician should pay particular attention to observing the knees for the following: signs of swelling, ecchymosis, deformity (increased varus/valgus, limited extension, hyperextension), and range of motion restrictions. Additionally, the ankle and foot mechanics should be noted in stance and with gait.

The examiner should observe the patient from the anterior, posterior, and lateral views.

Functional Tests

The patient should demonstrate any functional movement or activity that reproduces symptoms. These functional movements often include one or more of the followwing activities: walking, jogging, hopping, squatting, stepping up/down a step, transferring from sit to stand, and single leg standing.

These tests allow for a quick functional screen of the patient's entire lower quarter. Appropriate selection of the tests should be based on the patient's age, activity level, and severity of pain. The clinician should assess the quality and quantity of motion and any change in symptoms with test performance.

Palpation

The examiner palpates the knee region starting superficially and progressing to deeper structures. The examiner palpates for the presence of any temperature changes, moisture, soft tissue or lymph node swelling, and tissue texture abnormalities.

Depending on the patient history and the clinician's hypothesis of what regions are involved in the patient's pain or dysfunction, the clinician may also decide to palpate the hip, gluteal, and lumbo-sacral regions.

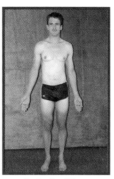
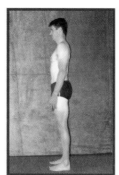
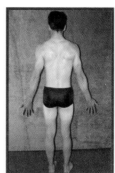

Anterior View   Lateral View   Posterior View

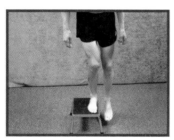
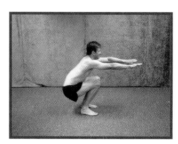

Functional Test: Step Down   Functional Test: Squat

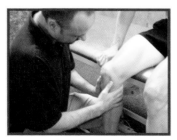
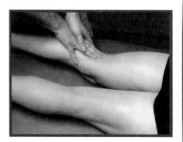

Anterior Knee   Posterior Knee

Knee

Active Range of Motion (AROM), Passive Range of Motion (PROM), & Overpressure:

With the patient supine, the examiner asks the patient to perform the following motions while assessing the quality and quantity of motion and change in symptoms. After performing active range of motion, the examiner passively moves the joint through maximal range of motion (as tolerated by the patient), applies overpressure, and assesses range of motion, pain reproduction, and end-feel. ROM can be quantified with a standard goniometer or gravity/bubble inclinometer.

Flexion

Supine: The patient is asked to bring the heel toward the buttock, bending the knee as far as possible. The examiner then flexes the knee through full passive range of motion. Overpressure can be applied at the end range of motion.

Extension

Supine: The patient is asked to straighten the knee as far as possible. The examiner then extends the knee through full passive extension range of motion. Overpressure can be applied at the end range of motion.

Note: The authors encourage examiners to include hip ROM assessment in a comprehensive knee examination. Refer to the Hip Chapter for more information.

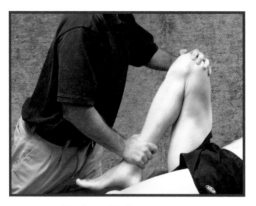

Flexion with Overpressure

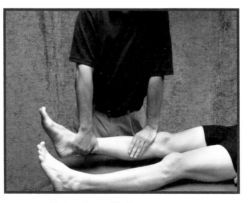

Extension with Overpressure

Resisted Muscle Tests:

Resisted tests are performed isometrically and are performed to assess symptom response & strength. The following table provides a list of selected resisted tests that should be performed when examining the knee.

Flexion in Sitting

Sitting: The examiner asks the patient to sit upright and to straighten the knee to approximately 20-30° knee flexion angle. While stabilizing the patient's distal thigh, the patient is then asked to resist examiner's downward (flexion) force that is applied to the patient's distal leg.

Extension in Sitting

Sitting: While stabilizing the patient's distal thigh, the patient is asked to resist examiner's extension force that is applied to the patient's distal leg. To apply the extension force, the examiner pulls on the distal leg with an anteriorly directed force.

Note: The authors encourage examiners to include hip resisted muscle tests (especially assessment of hip abduction and hip external rotation strength) in a comprehensive knee examination.

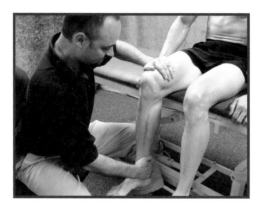

Resisted Flexion

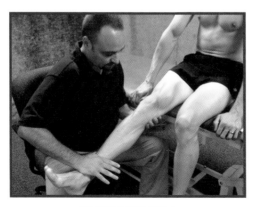

Resisted Extension

Knee

Muscle Length/Flexibility:

These tests are performed to assess the length and/or flexibility of the muscles that either directly or indirectly impact the knee if tight. Muscle length can often be quantified with a standard goniometer or gravity/bubble inclinometer.

Iliopsoas

Supine: Position the patient so that the buttocks and trunk are on the table. Flex the hips and knees until the lumbar spine is flat against the table. While maintaining the non-tested LE in this position, slowly lower the tested LE towards the floor by extending the hip. The final resting position of the hip can be measured to quantitatively assess iliopsoas muscle length. For normal length, the thigh should lie parallel to the treatment table, or fall below the level of the treatment table.

Prone: Stabilize the patient's ischeal tuberosity with one hand (apply posterior-to-anterior directed force) and passively extend the patient's hip with the other. You should be able to extend the hip at least 10°.

Rectus Femoris

Prone: Stabilize the patient's ischeal tuberosity with one hand (apply posterior-to-anterior directed force) and passively flex the patient's knee. Keep the hip in midline while performing this test, and don't allow either hip to flex.

Hamstrings

Supine: While keeping the non-tested LE stabilized against the table, flex hip of the tested LE to 90°. Have the patient help you maintain 90° hip flexion while you passively extend the knee. While no normative data is available, many determine that the hamstrings are tight if the patient lacks > 15-20° to reach full extension with this test.

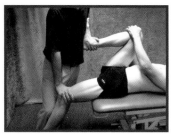

Iliopsoas in Supine

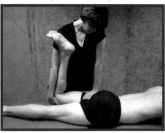

Iliopsoas in Prone

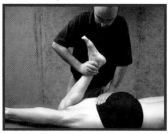

Rectus Femoris

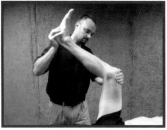

Hamstrings

Knee

Muscle Length/Flexibility Continued:

Tensor Fascia Latae and Iliotibial Band (Ober's Test)

Sidelying: Stabilize the patient's pelvis. Flex the bottom LE slightly to help stabilize the patient in sidelying. Flex the knee and hip of the tested LE (upper LE), passively abduct the hip, then extend the hip until the thigh is in line with the body. Keep the knee flexed to 90° while you lower the thigh. If the hip remains abducted (does not adduct beyond horizontal), then the patient has tightness of the TFL & ITB.

Gastrocnemius and Soleus

Supine: Passively dorsiflex the patient's ankle as far as possible and measure ankle dorsiflexion (DF). Perform test in full knee extension (assesses the gastrocnemius & soleus muscles) and in knee flexion (assesses the soleus muscle).

If the patient feels primarily a stretch or pull in the calf region, the examiner can feel more confident that the muscles are primarily limiting further ankle DF. If the patient feels pain or stiffness focused in the ankle is limiting further ankle DF, the examiner must conclude that a restriction in ankle DF range of motion (and not muscle length) is limiting the test.

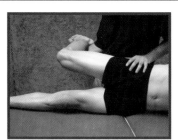

**Tensor Fascia Latae and
Iliotibial Band**

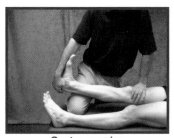

Gastrocnemius

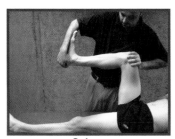

Soleus

Assessment of Accessory Movements:

The examiner investigates accessory movement of the knee with the patient in supine. With all accessory movement tests, pain responses are recorded, and mobility judgments are established as hypermobile, normal, or hypomobile.

Anterior Glide of the Tibia

Passively flex the knee to 90° and apply an anteriorly directed force to the proximal tibia.

Posterior Glide of the Tibia

Passively flex the knee to 90° and apply a posteriorly directed force to the proximal tibia.

Anterior and Posterior Glide of the Proximal Fibula

Passively flex the patient's knee approximately 90° and sit on the patient's toes to help stabilize the lower extremity. While using one hand to stabilize the proximal tibia, use the other hand to grasp the proximal fibula and apply a posteriorly (and slightly medial) directed force to assess anterior-to-posterior motion. Apply an anteriorly (and slightly lateral) force to assess posterior-to-anterior motion.

Patellar Glides

Passively flex the patient's knee approximately 30° and place it either over your knee or a bolster to keep it stable. Cup the patella with your more caudal hand (relative to the patient) to guide motion, and place the palm of your more cephalad hand over the base and anterior surface of the patella for force application. Apply an inferiorly directed force to the patella to assess inferior glide.

In order to assess superior patellar glide, simply reverse hand positions (your cephalad hand cups and guides motion of the patella while your caudad hand is placed over the apex and anterior patella for force application). Apply a superiorly directed force to the patella to assess superior glide.

With both inferior and superior glide assessment, be careful not to apply compressive force to the patella as this can easily aggravate symptoms. It is less likely that you will apply a compressive force to the patella if you crouch over and get your forearms in parallel with the plane of movement of the patella.

A medial glide to the patella is performed with the knee in full extension, glide the patella from lateral to medial to assess medial glide. Be sure to compare to the uninvolved lower extremity. This can also be performed in progressive degrees of knee flexion.

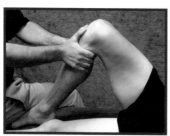

Anterior Glide of the Tibia

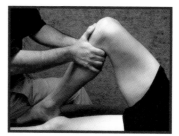

Posterior Glide of the Tibia

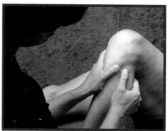

Anterior and Posterior Glides
of the Fibula

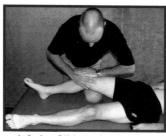

Inferior Glide to the Patella

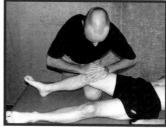

Superior Glide to the Patella

Knee

Special Tests:

Lachman Test

Purpose:
To test for the integrity of the anterior cruciate ligament (ACL).

Description:
The patient is supine and the tested LE is placed in approximately 20° knee flexion. The distal thigh should be stabilized, and the examiner attempts to translate the leg anteriorly on the stabilized femur.

There are several methods used by clinicians to stabilize the patient's distal thigh. The method shown here uses the examiner's thigh and hand for stabilization, while allowing the examiner to simultaneously palpate the joint line for tibial translation.

Positive Test:
The test result is considered to be positive if there is a lack of end point for tibial translation, or if there is excessive tibial translation.

Diagnostic Accuracy:[13-18]
Sensitivity = .65 - .99   - LR = 0.19 - 0.83
Specificity = .42 - .97   + LR = 1.12 - 27.3

Reliability:
For positive or negative findings.
Kappa = .19 (inter- examiner) to Kappa = .51 (intra-examiner).[14]
End-feel assessment ("hard" or "soft"), Kappa = .33 (intra- examiner).[14]

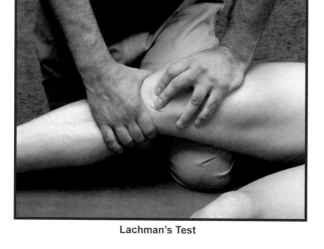

Lachman's Test

Anterior Drawer Test

Purpose:
To test the integrity of the anterior cruciate ligament (ACL).

Description:
The patient is supine and the tested LE is placed in approximately 90° knee flexion. The examiner sits on the patient's toes to help stabilize the LE. The examiner then grasps the proximal leg as shown and attempts to translate the leg anteriorly. By using the hand position shown with the thumbs placed over the joint line, the examiner is able to palpate the joint line for tibial translation.

Positive Test:
The test is considered positive if there is a lack of end point for tibial translation, or if there is excessive tibial translation.

Diagnostic Accuracy:[13,15-20]
Sensitivity = .41 - .91   - LR = .09 - .62
Specificity = .86 - 1.0   + LR = 5.4 - 8.2

Reliability:
For findings of normal or abnormal in patients with knee OA.
Kappa = .54 (inter- examiner).[4]

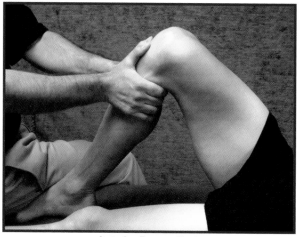

Anterior Drawer Test

Posterior Drawer Test

Purpose:
To test the integrity of the posterior cruciate ligament (PCL).

Description:
The patient is supine and the tested LE is placed in approximately 90° knee flexion. The examiner sits on the patient's toes to help stabilize the LE. The examiner then grasps the proximal leg as shown and attempts to translate the leg posteriorly. By using the hand position shown with the thumbs placed over the joint line, the examiner is able to palpate the joint line for tibial translation.

Positive Test:
The test result is considered to be positive if there is a lack of end point for tibial translation, or if there is excessive tibial translation.

Diagnostic Accuracy:[19]
Sensitivity = .90   - LR = .10
Specificity = .99   + LR = 90

Reliability:
For normal or abnormal findings.
Kappa = .82 (inter- examiner).[4]

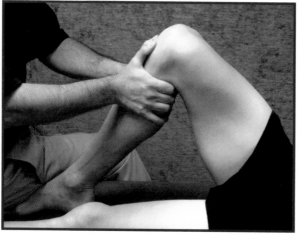

Posterior Drawer Test

Knee

Pivot-Shift Test

Purpose:
To test for the integrity of the anterior cruciate ligament (ACL)

Description:
The patient is supine and must be relaxed. The examiner lifts the LE keeping the knee fully extended. While applying a valgus stress, internal rotation force to the leg, and slight axial compression, the examiner slowly flexes the knee.

Positive Test:
The test result is considered to be positive if the lateral tibial plateau begins in an anteriorly subluxed position and shifts (or reduces) to a neutral position at about 30° knee flexion. This occurs because, at this point, the iliotibial band changes from a knee extender to a knee flexor, and the anterolateral tibial subluxation shifts, or reduces, back to a neutral position.

Diagnostic Accuracy:
Sensitivity = .71 - .90[15,16,18]   - LR = .18[15]
Specificity = .97 - .98[13,15]   + LR = 41[15]

Reliability:
Not reported

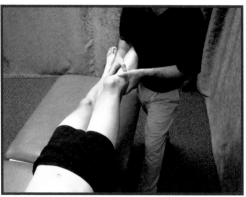

Pivot-Shift Test: Starting Position

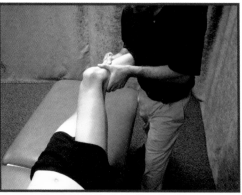

Pivot-Shift Test: Ending Position

Knee

Valgus Stress Test

Purpose:
To test the integrity of the tibial collateral ligament (TCL).*

Description:
The patient is supine and relaxed. The examiner lifts the LE and flexes the knee 20°- 30°. While palpating the medial joint line, the examiner applies a valgus force to the knee. The examiner should be careful to avoid simultaneously inducing rotary forces to the knee and hip.

Positive Test:
The test result is considered to be positive if pain or laxity are present.

Diagnostic Accuracy:
Sensitivity = .86 - .96[21,22]   - LR = NR
Specificity = NR   + LR = NR

Reliability:
For findings of normal or abnormal in patients with knee OA.

Kappa = .02 - .66 (inter- examiner). [4,23]

* Note: The TCL is also known as the medial collateral ligament, or MCL.

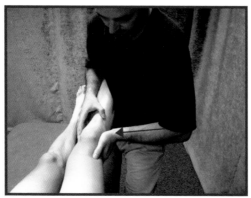

Valgus Stress Test Starting Position

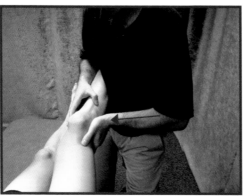

Valgus Stress Test Ending Position

Knee

Varus Stress Test

Purpose:
To test the integrity of the fibular collateral ligament (FCL).*

Description:
The patient is supine and relaxed. The examiner lifts the LE and flexes the knee 20°- 30°. While palpating the lateral joint line, the examiner applies a varus force to the knee. The examiner should be careful to avoid simultaneously inducing rotary forces to the knee and hip.

Positive Test:
The test result is considered to be positive if pain or laxity are present.

Diagnostic Accuracy:[22]
Sensitivity = .25   - LR = NR
Specificity = NR   + LR = NR

Reliability:
Inter-examiner reliability in patients with knee OA.
Kappa = 0.0 - .88.[4,23]

* Note: The FCL is also known as the lateral collateral ligament, or LCL

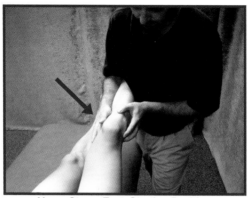

Varus Stress Test: Starting Position

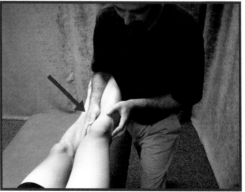

Varus Stress Test: Ending Position

McMurray Test

Purpose:
To test for the presence of a meniscus lesion.

Description:
The examiner flexes the hip and knee maximally, then applies a valgus force to the knee while externally rotating the leg and passively extending the knee completely. The maneuver is repeated from full flexion to full extension while internally rotating the leg and applying a varus force to the knee. The examiner should palpate the joint line while performing the test.*

Positive Test:
A palpable click or "thud", or provocation of pain.

Diagnostic Accuracy:[13,24-28]
Sensitivity = .16 - .95   - LR = .4 - 2.84
Specificity = .25 - 1.0   + LR = .39 - 11.6

Reliability:
Inter-examiner reliability in patients with knee OA:
Kappa = .16[23]

* Note that operational definitions for performance of this test, as well as definitions of a positive test, in the literature are quite variable.

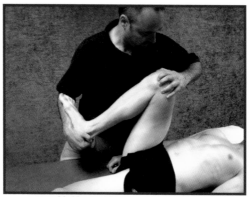

**McMurray Test: Valgus and
External Rotation Component**

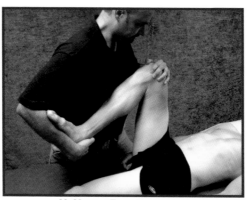

**McMurray Test: Varus and
Internal Rotation Component**

Knee

Joint Line Tenderness

Purpose:
To test for the presence of a meniscus lesion.

Description:
The examiner palpates the joint line of the knee. This is most often performed with the knee in 90° flexion.

Positive Test:
Provocation or reproduction of pain.

Diagnostic Accuracy: [13,25,27-30]
Sensitivity = .28 - .92   - LR = .08 - 2.53
Specificity = .29 - .97   + LR = .69 - 30.7

Reliability:
Kappa = .21 - .25[23]

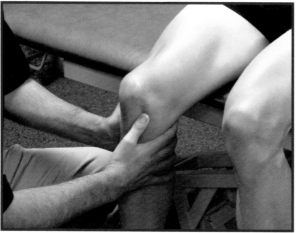

Palpation for Joint Line Tenderness

Knee

Special Tests:

Dynamic Test for Lateral Meniscus Lesions

Purpose:
To test for the presence of a lateral meniscus lesion.

Description:
With the patient in supine, position the hip at 60° abduction, flexed and externally rotated 45°, and the knee flexed 90°. The lateral border of the foot should rest on the examination table. Palpate the lateral joint line. While maintaining pressure over the lateral joint line, progressively adduct the hip while keeping a 90° knee flexion angle.

Positive Test:
The test is positive if:
   1) any pain that is present with pressure of the finger(s) over the joint line increases with hip adduction.
   2) sharp pain is felt when the final position is achieved.

Diagnostic Accuracy:
Sensitivity = .85   - LR = .17[31]
Specificity = .90   + LR = 8.5[31]

Reliability:
Kappa = .61 - .85[31]

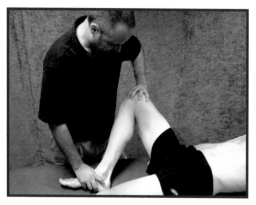

Dynamic Test Starting Position

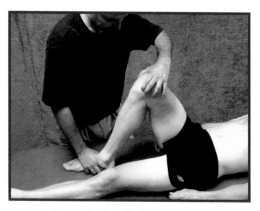

Dynamic Test Ending Position

Knee

Ottawa Knee Rules

Purpose:
To identify the need to order radiographs after knee trauma.

Description:
This is a clinical prediction rule. If one of the following variables is present, radiographs should be ordered:

1. Age > 55 years
2. Isolated patellar tenderness without other bone tenderness
3. Tenderness of the fibular head
4. Inability to flex to 90°
5. Inability to bear weight immediately after injury and in the emergency department (4 steps) regardless of limping.

Diagnostic Accuracy: [32-40]
Adult Population:
Sensitivity = 1.0   - LR = 0
Specificity = .49 - .56   + LR = 1.9 - 2.3

Pediatric Population:
Sensitivity = 1.0   - LR = 0
Specificity = .43   + LR = 1.8

Reliability:
Inter-examiner agreement for identification of predictor variables. Kappa= .77[34]

Clinical Diagnosis of Knee Osteoarthritis

Purpose:
To identify the presence of knee osteoarthritis (OA)

Description:
At least three of the following clinical criteria should be met to establish the diagnosis of knee OA:

1. Age > 50 years
2. Stiffness > 30 min
3. Crepitus
4. Bony tenderness
5. Bony enlargement
6. No palpable warmth

Diagnostic Accuracy:
Sensitivity = .95   − LR = .07[4]
Specificity = .69   + LR = 3.1[4]

Knee

Reference List

(1) Pecina MM, Bojanic I. Overuse Injuries of the Musculoskeletal System. Boca Raton: CRC Press; 1993.

(2) Fishman L, Dombi G, Michaelson C, Ringel S, Rozbruch J, Rosner B et al. Piriformis syndrome: Diagnosis, treatment and outcome- a 10-year study. *Arch Phys Med Rehabil* 2002; 83:295-301.

(3) Jones A, Hopkinson N, Pattrick M, Berman P, Doherty M. Evaluation of a method for clinically assessing osteoarthritis of the knee. *Ann Rheum Dis* 1992; 51(2):243-245.

(4) Cibere J, Bellamy N, Thorne A, Esdaile JM, McGorm KJ, Chalmers A et al. Reliability of the knee examination in osteoarthritis: effect of standardization. *Arthritis Rheum* 2004; 50(2):458-468.

(5) DeHaven KE. Diagnosis of acute knee injuries with hemarthrosis. *Am J Sports Med* 1980; 8(1):9-14.

(6) Greenfield B, Tovin B. Knee. Current Concpets in Orthopaedic Physical Therapy. La Crosse: Orthopaedic Section, American Physical Therapy Association; 2001.

(7) Hartley A. Practical Joint Assessment. St Louis: Mosby; 1995.

(8) Muellner T, Weinstabl R, Schabus R, Vecsei V, Kainberger F. The diagnosis of meniscal tears in athletes. A comparison of clinical and magnetic resonance imaging investigations. *Am J Sports Med* 1997; 25(1):7-12.

(9) Cook JL, Khan KM, Kiss ZS, Purdam CR, Griffiths L. Reproducibility and clinical utility of tendon palpation to detect patellar tendinopathy in young basketball players. Victorian Institute of Sport tendon study group. *Br J Sports Med* 2001; 35(1):65-69.

(10) Cleland J, McRae M. Patellofemoral pain syndrome: a critical analysis of current concepts. *Phys Ther Rev* 2002; 7:153-161.

(11) Grelsamer R, McConnell J. The Patella: A Team Approach. Gaithersburg: Aspen Publishers; 1998.

(12) Cassas KJ, Cassettari-Wayhs A. Childhood and adolescent sports-related overuse injuries. *Am Fam Physician* 2006; 73(6):1014-1022.

(13) Boeree NR, Ackroyd CE. Assessment of the menisci and cruciate ligaments: an audit of clinical practice. *Injury* 1991; 22(4):291-294.

(14) Cooperman JM, Riddle DL RJ. Reliability and validity of judgments of the integrity of the anterior cruciate ligament of the knee using the Lachman test. *Phys Ther* 1990; 70:225-233.

(15) Katz J, Fingeroth R. The diagnostic accurcy of ruptures of the anterior cruciate ligament comparing the Lachman test, the anterior drawer sign, and the pivot shift test in acute and chronic knee injuries. *Am J Sports Med* 1986; 14:88-91.

(16) Kim SJ, Kim HK. Reliability of the anterior drawer test, the pivot shift test, and the Lachman test. *Clin Orthop Relat Res* 1995;(317):237-242.

(17) Lee JK, Yao L, Phelps CT, Wirth CR, Czajka J, Lozman J. Anterior cruciate ligament tears: MR imaging compared with arthroscopy and clinical tests. *Radiology* 1988; 166(3):861-864.

(18) Liu SH, Osti L, Henry M, Bocchi L. The diagnosis of acute complete tears of the anterior cruciate ligament. Comparison of MRI, arthrometry and clinical examination. *J Bone Joint Surg Br* 1995; 77(4):586-588.

(19) Rubinstein RA, Jr., Shelbourne KD, McCarroll JR, et al. The accuracy of the clinical examination in the setting of posterior cruciate ligament injuries. *Am J Sports Med* 1994; 22(4):550-557.

(20) Braunstein EM. Anterior cruciate ligament injuries: a comparison of arthrographic and physical diagnosis. AJR Am J Roentgenol 1982; 138(3):423-425.

(21) Garvin GJ, Munk PL, Vellet AD. Tears of the medial collateral ligament: magnetic resonance imaging findings and associated injuries. *Can Assoc Radiol J* 1993; 44(3):199-204.

(22) Harilainen A. Evaluation of knee instability in acute ligamentous injuries. *Ann Chir Gynaecol* 1987; 76(5):269-273.

(23) Dervin GF, Stiell IG, Wells GA, et al. Physicians' accuracy and interrator reliability for the diagnosis of unstable meniscal tears in patients having osteoarthritis of the knee. *Can J Surg* 2001; 44(4):267-274.

Knee

(24) Anderson A, Lipscomb A. Clinical diagnosis of meniscal tears. Description of a new manipulative test. *Am J Sports Med* 1986; 14:291-293.

(25) Barry O, Smith H, McManus F, MacAuley P. Clinical assessment of suspected meniscal tears. *Ir J Med Sci* 1983; 152:149-151.

(26) Evans PJ, Bell GD, Frank C. Prospective evaluation of the McMurray test. *Am J Sports Med* 1993; 21(4):604-608.

(27) Fowler P, Lubliner JA. The predictive value of five clinical signs in the evaluation of meniscal pathology. *Arthroscopy* 1989; 5:184-186.

(28) Noble J, Erat K. In defence of the meniscus. A prospective study of 200 meniscectomy patients. *J Bone Joint Surg Br* 1980; 62-B(1):7-11.

(29) Eren OT. The accuracy of joint line tenderness by physical examination in the diagnosis of meniscal tears. *Arthroscopy* 2003; 19(8):850-854.

(30) Shelbourne KD, Martini DJ, McCarroll JR, VanMeter CD. Correlation of joint line tenderness and meniscal lesions in patients with acute anterior cruciate ligament tears. *Am J Sports Med* 1995; 23(2):166-169.

(31) Mariani PP, Adriani E, Maresca G, Mazzola CG. A prospective evaluation of a test for lateral meniscus tears. Knee Surg *Sports Traumatol Arthrosc* 1996; 4(1):22-26.

(32) Stiell IG, Wells GA, McDowell I, et al. Use of radiography in acute knee injuries: need for clinical decision rules. *Acad Emerg Med* 1995; 2(11):966-973.

(33) Stiell IG, Wells GA, McKnight RD. Validating the "real" Ottawa Knee Rule. *Ann Emerg Med* 1999; 33(2):241-243.

(34) Stiell IG, Wells GA, Hoag RH, et al. Implementation of the Ottawa Knee Rule for the use of radiography in acute knee injuries. *JAMA* 1997; 278(23):2075-2079.

(35) Stiell IG, Greenberg GH, Wells GA, et al. Prospective validation of a decision rule for the use of radiography in acute knee injuries. *JAMA* 1996; 275(8):611-615.

(36) Stiell IG, Greenberg GH, Wells GA, et al. Derivation of a decision rule for the use of radiography in acute knee injuries. *Ann Emerg Med* 1995; 26(4):405-413.

(37) Bulloch B, Neto G, Plint A, et al. Validation of the Ottawa Knee Rule in children: a multicenter study. *Ann Emerg Med* 2003; 42(1):48-55.

(38) Khine H, Dorfman DH, Avner JR. Applicability of Ottawa knee rule for knee injury in children. *Pediatr Emerg Care* 2001; 17(6):401-404.

(39) Ketelslegers E, Collard X, Vande BB, et al. Validation of the Ottawa knee rules in an emergency teaching centre. *Eur Radiol* 2002; 12(5):1218-1220.

(40) Bachmann LM, Haberzeth S, Steurer J, et al. The accuracy of the Ottawa knee rule to rule out knee fractures: a systematic review. *Ann Intern Med 2004*; 140(2):121-124.

(41) Altman RD. Criteria for classification of clinical osteoarthritis. *J Rheumatol Suppl* 1991; 27:10-12.

Knee

FOOT AND ANKLE EXAMINATION

In This Chapter:

1. **Historical Examination & Referral Patterns**
2. **Observation, Functional Quick Tests, and Palpation**
3. **Active Range of Motion, Passive Range of Motion, and Overpressure**
    a. Dorsiflexion & Plantar Flexion
    b. Inversion and Eversion
4. **Resisted Muscle Tests**
    a. Dorsiflexion & Plantar Flexion
    b. Inversion and Eversion
5. **Muscle & Tissue Length/Flexibility**
    a. Gastrocnemius & Soleus
    b. Plantar Fascia
6. **Assessment of Accessory Movements**
    a. Anterior to Posterior Glide & Posterior to Anterior Glide of the Talus
    b. Anterior to Posterior Glide & Posterior to Anterior Glide of the Distal Fibula
    c. Subtalar Joint Inversion/Eversion
7. **Special Tests**
    a. Anterior Drawer
    b. Talar Tilt
    c. Anterior Impingement Sign
    d. Squeeze Test & External Rotation Test
    e. Calf Squeeze Test
    f. Navicular Drop Test
    g. Ottawa Ankle Rules

Foot
& Ankle

Region Specific Historical Examination:

In addition to the historical examination presented in Chapter three, the patient should be asked specific questions related to the leg, ankle, and foot, and proximal surrounding regions.

1. *Do your symptoms change (better or worse) with any movements of the low back? Do you have any pain in your low back, even if you feel it is unrelated to your leg/ankle/foot pain?*

   If the patient answers "yes" for either question, the lumbopelvic region and hip should be examined in addition to the leg, ankle, and/or foot.

2. *Does your foot/ankle pain extend up into your knee, thigh, hip, or back? Do you ever experience numbness or tingling into the hip, thigh, leg, ankle, or foot?*

   If the patient answers "yes" for any question, both a LE neurological screening examination and a lumbar spine examination should be performed to identify any existing radiculopathy or radiculitis.

   If symptoms are reported in the posterior thigh and perhaps the calf, but no numbness/tingling, the following diagnoses should be considered: Ischial bursitis[1], Hamstring strain[1], and piriformis syndrome.[2]

3. *Have you recently increased your physical activity, especially running (distance, terrain, speed) or other weight-bearing activities?*

   If the patient answers "yes" the clinician should be suspicious of a femoral, tibial, or fibular or metatarsal stress reaction or stress fracture. Muscle sprain/strain should also be considered.

4. *Do you have ankle pain or stiffness that eases after a few hours in the morning?*

   If the patient answers "yes" the clinician should be suspicious of knee osteoarthritis.[3,4]

5. **Do you have pain in the bottom of your foot that is worse when you initially bear weight (especially in the morning), and also worsens with prolonged time up on your feet?**

> If the patient answers "yes" the clinician should be suspicious of plantar fasciitis/fasciosis and/or calcaneal heel spur.

6. **Is your leg, ankle, or foot pain a result of trauma, such as injury with jumping/landing, changing directions with your foot planted, or twisting?**

> If the patient answers "yes" the following diagnoses should be considered: ligamentous injury, talar dome osteochondral defect, fracture, ankle sprain.[5-8]

> If the injury described resulted in an eversion, external rotation, and/or dorsiflexion force to the ankle, the clinician should be suspicious of syndesmosis injury, fracture, and talar dome injury (such as osteochondral defect).

7. **Have you ever had, or do you presently have active cancer, paralysis, paresis, recent plaster immobilization, recent period of bedrest, localized tenderness over the deep venous system, lower leg swelling, pitting edema, or collateral superficial veins?**

> If the patient answers "yes" consider using the clinical decision rule established by Wells and colleagues[9] to identify deep vein thrombosis.

8. **Do you or have you had a sudden episode of redness, heat, swelling, and pain? Have you recently consumed greater than normal portions of meats, seafood, beans, or other foods high in purines? Increased intake of alcohol?**

> If the patient answers "yes" consider gout as a possible diagnosis. A definitive diagnosis is established by finding uric acid crystals in the joint fluid during a gout attack.

Foot & Ankle

Observation, Functional Quick Tests, and Palpation:

Observation

Watch the patient walk and observe any abnormal gait mechanics and/or reproduction of symptoms.

With the patient standing, the examiner observes for any asymmetries in any of the soft tissues or bony landmarks of the hip, gluteal region, low back, and lower extremities. The examiner should observe the patient from the anterior, posterior, and lateral views.

Functional Tests

The patient should demonstrate any functional movement or activity that reproduces symptoms. These functional movements often include one or more of the following activities: walking, jogging, hopping, squatting, donning/doffing socks and shoes, transferring from sit to stand, single leg stance, and going up and down steps.

These tests allow for a quick functional screen of the patient's entire lower quarter. Appropriate selection of the tests should be based on the patient's age, activity level, and severity of pain. The clinician should assess the quality and quantity of motion and any change in symptoms with test performance.

Palpation

The examiner palpates the leg, ankle, and foot regions starting superficially and progressing to deeper structures. The examiner palpates for the presence of any temperature changes, moisture, soft tissue swelling, and tissue texture abnormalities. Additionally, the examiner should palpate for pulses over the dorsalis pedis artery and the posterior tibial artery.

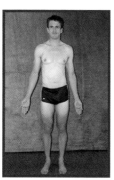
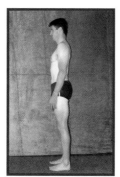
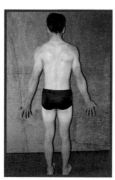

Anterior View   **Lateral View**   **Posterior View**

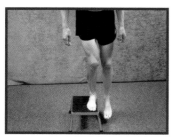

**Functional Test:
Step Down**

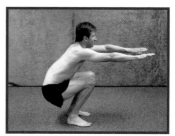

**Functional Test:
Squat**

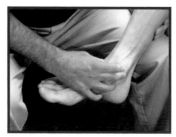

Palpation

Foot
& Ankle

Active Range of Motion (AROM), Passive Range of Motion (PROM), and Overpressure:

With the patient in sitting or in supine, the examiner asks the patient to perform the following motions while assessing the quality and quantity of motion and change in symptoms. After performing active range of motion, the examiner passively moves the joint through maximal range of motion (as tolerated by the patient), applies overpressure, and assesses range of motion, pain reproduction, and end-feel. ROM can be quantified with a standard goniometer or gravity/bubble inclinometer.

Dorsiflexion and Plantar Flexion

The patient is asked pull the toes and foot upwards toward the head. While maintaining the ankle in a neutral rotation, without allowing ankle inversion or eversion, the clinician moves the ankle through full passive dorsiflexion range of motion. Overpressure can be applied at the end range of motion.

Next, the patient is asked to point the toes, causing ankle plantarflexion.. This will cause the patient to plantar flex his ankle. The clinician then moves the ankle through full passive plantar flexion range of motion. Overpressure can be applied at the end range of motion.

Inversion and Eversion

The patient is asked to invert the foot. Cues from the clinician can include visual cues (showing the patient how to move the foot), verbal cues ("turn your foot inward as if you were trying to look at the bottom of the foot"), etc. The clinician then moves the ankle through full inversion. Overpressure can be applied at the end range of motion.

Next, the patient is asked to evert the foot, or turn the foot outward. The clinician then moves the ankle through full eversion. Overpressure can be applied at the end range of motion.

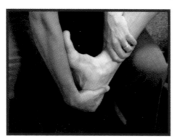

Dorsiflexion with Overpressure

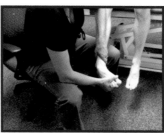

Plantar Flexion with Overpressure

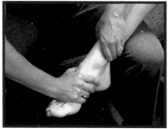

Inversion with Overpressure

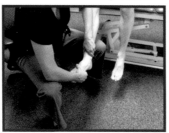

Eversion with Overpressure

Resisted Muscle Tests:

Resisted tests are performed isometrically and are performed to assess symptom response and strength. The following list provides selected resisted tests that should be performed when examining the leg, ankle, and foot region. Tests can be performed with the patient in sitting, supine, or prone. Tests will be shown here with the patient in a seated position.

Dorsiflexion and Plantar Flexion

The patient is asked pull the toes and foot upwards toward the head. The clinician should allow slight inversion with this motion. While stabilizing the patient's leg, the patient is asked to resist and inferiorly directed force produced by the examiner downward through the distal half of the foot. Additionally, a slight eversion force should be applied. This test will preferentially test the tibialis anterior muscle.

Next, the patient is asked to point the toes, causing ankle plantarflexion. This will cause the patient to plantar flex his ankle. While stabilizing the patient's leg, the patient is asked to resist an upwardly directed force produced by the examiner through the distal half of the foot. Note that only substantial weakness in plantar flexion strength will be detected with a manual muscle test. Single leg heel raises (the patient repeatedly lifts up onto the toes while in single leg stance) will challenge the plantar flexion musculature more appropriately for patients with normal or close to normal strength.

Inversion and Eversion

The patient is asked to invert the foot and point the toes downwards slightly to get the foot positioned into a combined position of inversion and plantar flexion. Cues from the clinician can include visual cues (showing the patient how to move the foot), verbal cues ("turn your foot inwards as if you were trying to look at the bottom of the foot"), etc. While stabilizing the leg, the clinician then asks the patient to resist force applied in an upward (dorsiflexion) and outward (eversion) direction. This test will preferentially test the tibialis longus muscle and other key muscles that plantarflex and invert the ankle.

Next, the patient is asked to evert the foot, or turn the foot outward, and point downwards slightly to get the foot positioned into a combined position of eversion and plantar flexion. While stabilizing the leg, the clinician then asks the patient to resist force applied in an upward (dorsiflexion) and inward (inversion) position. This test will preferentially test the fibularis longus and brevis.

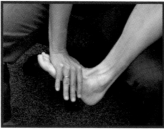

Resisted Dorsiflexion

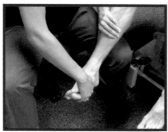

Resisted Plantarflexion

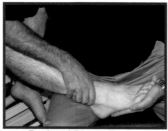

Resisted Inversion

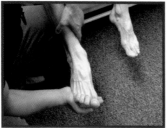

Resisted Eversion

Muscle Length/Flexibility:

These tests are performed to assess the length and/or flexibility of the ankle, leg, and associated tissues. The following table provides a list of selected resisted tests that should be performed when examining this region. Muscle length can often be quantified with a standard goniometer or gravity/bubble inclinometer.

Gastrocnemius and Soleus

Supine: Passively dorsiflex the patient's ankle as far as possible and measure ankle dorsiflexion (DF). Perform the test in full knee extension (assesses the gastrocnemius and soleus muscles) and in knee flexion (assesses the soleus muscle).

If the patient feels a stretch or pull in the calf or Achilles tendon region, the examiner can feel more confident that the muscles are primarily limiting further ankle DF. If the patient feels pain or stiffness in the ankle is limiting further ankle DF, the examiner should conclude that a joint restriction in ankle DF range of motion, and not muscle length, may be the primary factor limiting DF range of motion.

Plantar Fascia

The clinician passively dorsiflexes the patient's ankle and, while maintaining ankle dorsiflexion, extends the toes. This test should be performed with the knee in flexion to minimize the stretch to the gastrocnemius muscle.

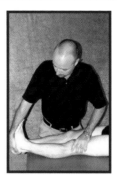

Gastrocnemius

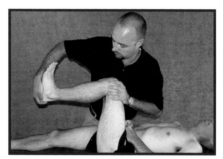

Soleus

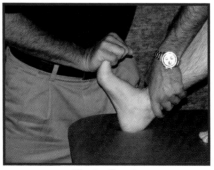

Plantar Fascia

Foot
& Ankle

Assessment of Accessory Movements

The examiner investigates accessory movement of the ankle joint in supine and prone. With all tests, pain responses are recorded and mobility judgments are established as hypermobile, normal, or hypomobile.

Posterior to Anterior Glide of the Talus

Supine/sitting: With the patient's foot draped just off the edge of the plinth, the clinician will stabilize the anterior distal leg with one hand. Use the other hand to grasp the posterior talus and rearfoot and move the talus/rearfoot anteriorly on the stabilized leg.

Anterior to Posterior Glide of the Talus

Supine/sitting: With the patient's foot draped just off the edge of the plinth, the clinician will stabilize the posterior distal leg with one hand. Use the other hand to grasp the talus and move the foot/talus posteriorly on the stabilized lower leg.

Anterior to Posterior Glides of the Distal Fibula

Supine/sitting: With the patient's heel draped just off the edge of the plinth, the clinician will stabilize the distal tibia with one hand. Grasp the end of the fibula with the thenar eminence of the other hand and move the distal fibula posteriorly on the stabilized tibia.

Posterior to Anterior Glides of the Distal Fibula

Supine/sitting: As above, except the clinician will now stabilize the distal fibula with one hand, grasp the end of the tibia with the other hand, and move the distal tibia posteriorly on the stabilized fibula.

Prone, with the patient's foot draped just off the edge of the plinth, the clinician will stabilize the distal tibia with one hand. Grasp the end of the fibula with the thenar eminence of the other hand and move the distal fibula anteriorly on the stabilized tibia.

Subtalar Joint

Sitting, with the patient in sitting with the foot draped just off the edge of the plinth, the clinician stabilizes the distal leg with one hand and use the other hand to grasp the calcaneus with the ankle positioned in neutral. The clinician then passively moves the rearfoot into inversion and into eversion.

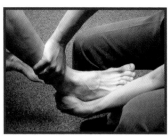

Anterior Glide of Talus

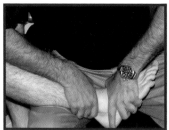

Posterior Glide of Talus

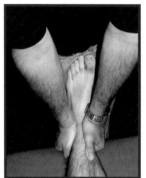

Posterior Glide to Fibula

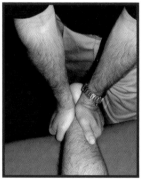

Anterior Glide to Fibula

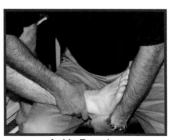

Ankle Eversion

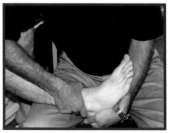

Ankle Inversion

Foot
& Ankle

Special Tests:

Anterior Drawer

Purpose:
To test for ligamentous laxity of the ankle (predominately tests anterior talofibular ligament).

Description:
The patient is in sitting or supine. The distal leg is stabilized anteriorly. The clinician grasps the patient's rearfoot, positions the ankle in 10-15 degrees plantar flexion, and translates ("draws") the rearfoot anteriorly.

Positive Test:
The test result is considered to be positive if the talus translates or subluxes anteriorly. It is often graded on a 4-point scale, ranging from "0" indicating no laxity to "3" indicating gross laxity.

Diagnostic Accuracy:
Acute testing (<48 hrs after injury):
Sensitivity = 0.71   - LR = 0.88[10]
Specificity = 0.33   + LR = 1.06[10]

Reliability:
Not reported

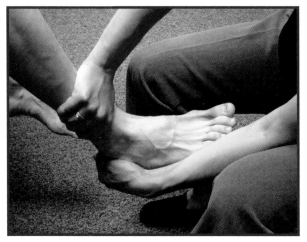

Anterior Drawer Test

Talar Tilt

Purpose:
To test for injury of the lateral ankle ligaments.

Description:
The patient is in sitting or supine. The distal leg is stabilized and the ankle is inverted. The clinician determines the amount of inversion.

Positive Test:
The amount of ankle laxity is used to grade the test. A 4-point scale, ranging from "0" indicating no laxity to "3" indicating gross laxity. An alternative method for grading is based on the degrees of inversion (<5 deg, 5-15 deg, >15 deg).

Diagnostic Accuracy:
Under general anesthetic, ≥ 15° inversion, or tilt, was always associated with complete anterior talofibular ligament and calcaneofibular ligament rupture.[12]

Reliability:
Not reported

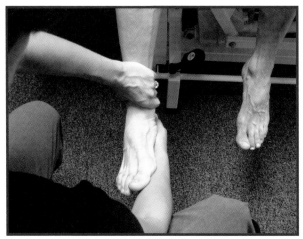

Talar Tilt Test

Impingement Sign

Purpose:
To test for anterior impingement at the talocrural joint.

Test One:

Description:
With the patient seated, the clinician grasps the calcaneus with one hand and uses the other hand to grasp the forefoot and bring it into plantarflexion. Then the examiner places the thumb over the anterolateral ankle. While maintaining pressure over the anterolateral ankle, the foot is then brought from plantarflexion to dorsiflexion.

Positive Test:
If pain is provoked with pressure from the examiner's thumb, and the pain is greater in dorsiflexion than in plantarflexion, then the test is positive.

Diagnostic Accuracy:
Sensitivity = .95   - LR = .06[13]
Specificity = .88   + LR = 7.9[13]

Reliability:
Not Reported

Test Two:

Description:
Record aggravating factors and loss of motion. Examination includes observation of swelling, passive forced ankle dorsiflexion and eversion, AROM, and double and single leg squats.

Positive Test:
The test is positive if ≥ 5 of the following findings are positive:
    1. Anterolateral ankle joint tenderness.
    2. Anterolateral ankle joint swelling.
    3. Pain with forced dorsiflexion and eversion.
    4. Pain with single leg squat.
    5. Pain with activities.
    6. Ankle instability.

Diagnostic Accuracy:
Sensitivity = .94   - LR = .08[14]
Specificity = .75   + LR = 3.8[14]

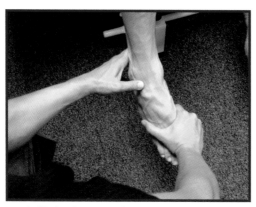

Ankle Impingement Test: Starting Position

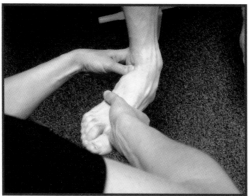

Ankle Impingement Test: Ending Position

Squeeze & External Rotation Tests

Purpose:
Both tests are for identifying tibiofibular syndesmotic injuries.

Squeeze Test

Description:
The patient is supine. Compress and release the tibia and fibula together midway up the calf.

Positive Test:
If pain is provoked in the area of the syndesmosis, the test is positive.

Reliability:
Kappa = .5[15]

External Rotation Test

Description:
The patient is supine or seated. The examiner maintains ankle dorsiflexion and externally rotates the foot on a stabilized leg.

Positive Test:
If pain is provoked in the area of the syndesmosis (anterior or posterior), or over the interosseous membrane, the test is positive.

Reliability:
Kappa = .75[15]

Diagnostic Accuracy (both tests)[16]
Values not reported. However, a relationship existed between confirmed diagnosis of syndesmosis through arthroscopic visualization and the squeeze test (p=0.02) and the ER test (p=0.03).

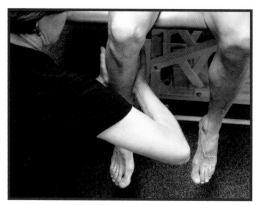

Squeeze Test

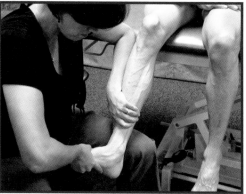

External Rotation Test

Calf Squeeze Test

Purpose:
To detect Achilles Tendon ruptures or tears.

Description:
With the patient in prone, gently squeeze the calf.

Positive Test:
The ankle remains still, or there is minimal plantarflexion relative to the other side.

Diagnostic Accuracy: [17,18]
Sensitivity = .96   - LR = .04
Specificity = .93   + LR = 13.7

Reliability:
Not reported

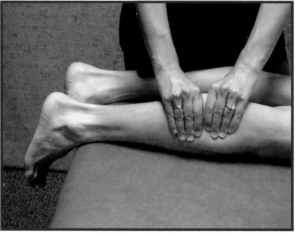

Calf Squeeze Test

Navicular Drop Test

Purpose:
A measurement of navicular height.

Description:
Mark the navicular tuberosity. Measure navicular height with the patient in subtalar neutral position with most weight on the contralateral lower extremity. Measure again maintaining the patient in relaxed bilateral stance and full weight-bearing. The difference between these two measurements is the navicular drop.

Reliability:[19-23]
Intra-examiner: .33 - .90
Inter-examiner: .31 - .74

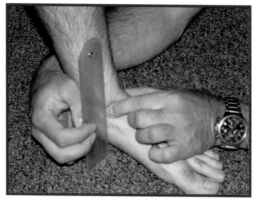

Navicular Drop Test: Measurement in Subtalar Neutral

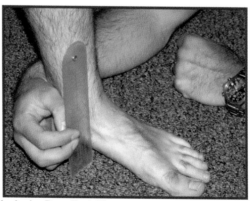

Navicular Drop Test: Measurement in Relaxed Stance

Foot
& Ankle

Ottawa Ankle Rules

Purpose
To determine the need to order radiographs after acute ankle injury.

Refer for radiographs:
If there is pain in the malleolar or midfoot area, and any one of the following:

An inability to bear weight both immediately after injury and in the emergency department for four steps.

Bone tenderness along any of the following areas:
- the distal 6 cm of the posterior edge of the tibia or tip of the medial malleolus
- the distal 6 cm of the posterior edge of the fibula or tip of the lateral malleolus
- the base of the fifth metatarsal (for foot injuries), or the navicular bone (for foot injuries).

Diagnostic Accuracy (pooled from 27 studies)[24]
Sensitivity = .98   - LR = .10

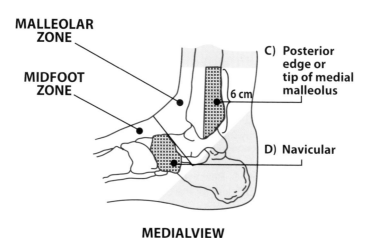

A) Posterior edge or tip of lateral malleolus

6 cm

B) Base of 5th Metatarsal

MALLEOLAR ZONE

MIDFOOT ZONE

LATERAL VIEW

MALLEOLAR ZONE

MIDFOOT ZONE

C) Posterior edge or tip of medial malleolus

6 cm

D) Navicular

MEDIAL VIEW

Used with permission from Stiell, I. et al. BMJ 1995;311:594-597

Foot & Ankle

Reference List

(1) Pecina MM, Bojanic I. Overuse Injuries of the Musculoskeletal System. Boca Raton: CRC Press; 1993.

(2) Fishman L, Dombi G, Michaelson C, et al. Piriformis syndrome: Diagnosis, treatment and outcome- a 10-year study. *Arch Phys Med Rehabil* 2002; 83:295-301.

(3) Jones A, Hopkinson N, Pattrick M, et al. Evaluation of a method for clinically assessing osteoarthritis of the knee. *Ann Rheum Dis* 1992; 51(2):243-245.

(4) Cibere J, Bellamy N, Thorne A, et al. Reliability of the knee examination in osteoarthritis: effect of standardization. *Arthritis Rheum* 2004; 50(2):458-468.

(5) DeHaven KE. Diagnosis of acute knee injuries with hemarthrosis. *Am J Sports Med* 1980; 8(1):9-14.

(6) Greenfield B, Tovin B. Knee. Current Concpets in Orthopaedic Physical Therapy. La Crosse: Orthopaedic Section, American Physical Therapy Association; 2001.

(7) Hartley A. Practical Joint Assessment. St Louis: Mosby; 1995.

(8) Muellner T, Weinstabl R, Schabus R, et al. The diagnosis of meniscal tears in athletes. A comparison of clinical and magnetic resonance imaging investigations. *Am J Sports Med* 1997; 25(1):7-12.

(9) Wells PS, Anderson DR, Bormanis J, et al. Value of assessment of pretest probability of deep-vein thrombosis in clinical management. *Lancet* 1997; 350(9094):1795-1798.

(10) van Dijk CN, Mol BW, Lim LS, et al. Diagnosis of ligament rupture of the ankle joint. Physical examination, arthrography, stress radiography and sonography compared in 160 patients after inversion trauma. *Acta Orthop Scand* 1996; 67(6):566-570.

(11) van Dijk CN, Lim LS, Bossuyt PM, Marti RK. Physical examination is sufficient for the diagnosis of sprained ankles. *J Bone Joint Surg Br* 1996; 78(6):958-962.

(12) Gaebler C, Kukla C, Breitenseher MJ, et al. Diagnosis of lateral ankle ligament injuries. Comparison between talar tilt, MRI and operative findings in 112 athletes. *Acta Orthop Scand* 1997; 68(3):286-290.

(13) Molloy S, Solan MC, Bendall SP. Synovial impingement in the ankle. A new physical sign. *J Bone Joint Surg Br* 2003; 85(3):330-333.

(14) Liu SH, Nuccion SL, Finerman G. Diagnosis of anterolateral ankle impingement. Comparison between magnetic resonance imaging and clinical examination. *Am J Sports Med* 1997; 25(3):389-393.

(15) Alonso A, Khoury L, Adams R. Clinical tests for ankle syndesmosis injury: reliability and prediction of return to function. *J Orthop Sports Phys Ther* 1998; 27(4):276-284.

(16) Beumer A, Swierstra BA, Mulder PG. Clinical diagnosis of syndesmotic ankle instability: evaluation of stress tests behind the curtains. *Acta Orthop Scand* 2002; 73(6):667-669.

(17) Maffulli N. The clinical diagnosis of subcutaneous tear of the Achilles tendon. A prospective study in 174 patients. *Am J Sports Med* 1998; 26(2):266-270.

(18) Maffulli N, Kenward MG, Testa V, et al. Clinical diagnosis of Achilles tendinopathy with tendinosis. *Clin J Sport Med* 2003; 13(1):11-15.

(19) Picciano AM, Rowlands MS, Worrell T. Reliability of open and closed kinetic chain subtalar joint neutral positions and navicular drop test. *J Orthop Sports Phys Ther 1993; 18(4):553-558.*

(20) Saltzman CL, Nawoczenski DA, Talbot KD. Measurement of the medial longitudinal arch. *Arch Phys Med Rehabil* 1995; 76(1):45-49.

(21) Sell KE, Verity TM, Worrell TW, Pease BJ, Wigglesworth J. Two measurement techniques for assessing subtalar joint position: a reliability study. *J Orthop Sports Phys Ther 1994*; 19(3):162-167.

(22) Vinicombe A, Raspovic A, Menz HB. Reliability of navicular displacement measurement as a clinical indicator of foot posture. *J Am Podiatr Med Assoc* 2001; 91(5):262-268.

(23) Menz HB, Tiedemann A, Kwan MM, et al. Reliability of clinical tests of foot and ankle characteristics in older people. *J Am Podiatr Med Assoc* 2003; 93(5):380-387.

(24) Bachmann LM, Kolb E, Koller MT, et al. Accuracy of Ottawa ankle rules to exclude fractures of the ankle and mid-foot: systematic review. *BMJ* 2003; 326(7386):417.

Foot & Ankle

INDEX

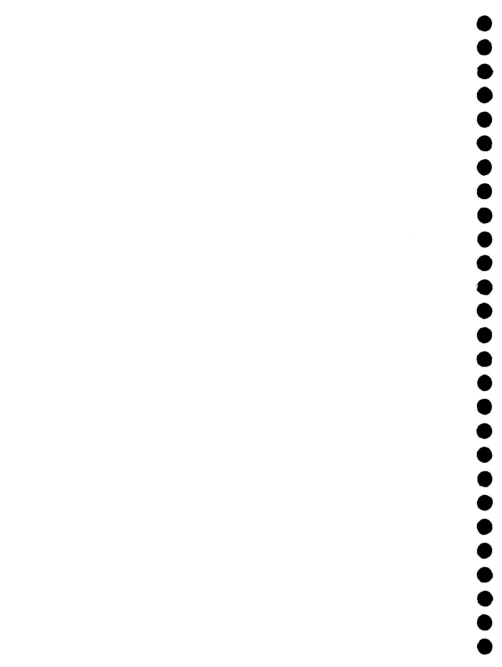